MATHEMATICS
EXPLAINED
for HEALTHCARE
PRACTITIONERS

DEREK HAYLOCK
& PAUL WARBURTON

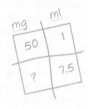

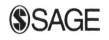SAGE

Los Angeles | London | New Delhi
Singapore | Washington DC

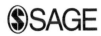

Los Angeles | London | New Delhi
Singapore | Washington DC

SAGE Publications Ltd
1 Oliver's Yard
55 City Road
London EC1Y 1SP

SAGE Publications Inc.
2455 Teller Road
Thousand Oaks, California 91320

SAGE Publications India Pvt Ltd
B 1/I 1 Mohan Cooperative Industrial Area
Mathura Road
New Delhi 110 044

SAGE Publications Asia-Pacific Pte Ltd
3 Church Street
#10-04 Samsung Hub
Singapore 049483

Editor: Susan Worsey
Assistant Editor: Emma Milman
Production editor: Katie Forsythe
Copyeditor: Rosemary Campbell
Proofreader: Beth Crockett
Marketing manager: Tamara Navaratnam
Cover design: Wendy Scott
Typeset by: C&M Digitals (P) Ltd, Chennai, India
Printed by MPG Books Group, Bodmin, Cornwall

Library of Congress Control Number: 2012939023

British Library Cataloguing in Publication data

A catalogue record for this book is available from
the British Library

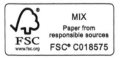

ISBN 978-1-4462-1118-2
ISBN 978-1-4462-1119-9 (pbk)

CONTENTS

About the Authors   vi

Acknowledgements   vii

Introduction   viii

A Disclaimer   xii

1   Understanding the Number System   1

2   Addition and Subtraction Skills   15

3   Multiplication and Division Skills   28

4   Units of Length   49

5   Units of Liquid Volume   57

6   Units of Weight   64

7   Using a Calculator   72

8   Rounding   83

9   Calculations with Decimal Numbers   98

10 Imperial Units Still in Use   115

11 Understanding Fractions and Ratios   127

12 Proportionality and 'Per'   145

13 Percentages   165

14 Miscellaneous Mathematics   183

15 Application   202

Answers to Check-ups   223

Index   244

ABOUT THE AUTHORS

Derek Haylock is an education consultant and author. He is a Senior Fellow at the University of East Anglia, Norwich, where he worked for over 30 years in teacher education. He is internationally known for his research and writing in the field of mathematics education; his work in mathematics education has taken him to Germany, Belgium, Lesotho, Kenya, Brunei and India. Derek is a major author in mathematics education, with a large number of published books and chapters in books. His best-selling book *Mathematics Explained for Primary Teachers* (Sage Publications) has been the leader in the field for many years, with a fourth edition published in 2010. His work is characterized by a commitment to explain mathematics in simple and accessible ways and to enable children and adults to learn the subject with understanding and confidence.

Paul Warburton is a registered nurse, senior lecturer and the coordinator of the Non-Medical Prescribing (NMP) programme at Edge Hill University, Ormskirk, Lancashire. Paul was also the project leader for the development and implementation of the NHS North-West Strategic Health Authority's on-line Numeracy Assessment Tool. Paul developed his interest in the numeracy skills of healthcare practitioners when he noted the incidence of qualified and even senior healthcare practitioners failing the NMP programme because of poor numeracy. He has extensive experience of writing and conference presentation about numeracy, non-medical prescribing and patient safety.

ACKNOWLEDGEMENTS

We wish especially to thank Susan Worsey of Sage Publications for bringing us together to write this book and for her encouragement and advice. Derek wishes to acknowledge the contribution of his wife, Christina, both for her support during the long months that he has spent at the top of the house working on this book and for her help in checking the final manuscript. Paul wishes to thank Nora, Michael and Rachel for their patience, support and understanding during the writing of this book.

INTRODUCTION

Welcome to this book on mathematics in healthcare practice and, assuming you have, well done in deciding to read the introduction! It is likely that you have picked up this book because you are working or training in some area of healthcare and have some concern about your personal confidence in the aspects of numeracy that are required in your professional work or training. You may be keen to learn more about the applications of mathematical understanding and skills in healthcare practice; or you may just be looking to revise and improve your own skills. Whatever the reason, we hope that your engagement with this book will prove to be an important step on the journey to improved mathematical skills, knowledge and understanding.

Why is this book needed?

The book is written for both qualified and pre-registration healthcare practitioners, whatever their chosen profession, and contains information, explanation, exercises and advice that will enable you, the reader, to improve your numeracy skills in practice. Our aim is also that you will develop an *understanding* of the underpinning mathematical processes and concepts involved. We appreciate that there is a risk that your enthusiasm to continue reading may now start to decline, but we really do want to help the reader to learn with understanding, not just to learn rules and recipes that make little sense to them. We recognize that many people are challenged by the numerical demands that occur in professional practice and become anxious when people start talking about 'mathematics', 'numeracy' or 'calculation'. Our aim is to replace that anxiety with confidence, the kind of confidence that is based on some degree of understanding of what is going on when we use and manipulate numbers. We hope that even those practitioners who start out with deeply-embedded feelings of anxiety and insecurity about mathematics will find the content and style of the book to be accessible, relevant, interesting, stimulating, and even enjoyable.

The material that we cover here is selected to enable practitioners to deal confidently and competently with the calculations and numerical situations that they will encounter on a daily basis in their work. Recognizing the importance of understanding, we encourage the reader to develop mental strategies for handling calculations, to draw upon their existing knowledge, to check that answers make sense and to develop a feeling for numbers and the relationships they have with each other. Throughout the book examples of calculations are taken, where appropriate, from a healthcare context to explain the mathematical ideas and to illustrate how the calculations are performed in practice.

Accuracy in numeracy skills and understanding of numbers are important life skills that are needed by everyone to cope confidently with a range of everyday situations such as shopping, working out the cost of utility bills, how much money is left in a bank account and dividing a pizza fairly. In a healthcare setting there are specific numeracy skills that are essential to enable practitioners to deal accurately and confidently with such things as drug doses, infusion rates, body mass indices and patient fluid balances. In everyday life mediocre or low numeracy skills may cause occasional embarrassment or even leave a person open to exploitation by others. But in a healthcare setting the consequences of poor numeracy skills can be serious not just for the practitioner but also for their patients. Patients have the right to expect that healthcare professionals are competent in the calculations that relate to their care and treatment. However, there is evidence from studies in the United Kingdom and elsewhere that inadequate levels of numeracy amongst healthcare practitioners is not uncommon, and that some health-care staff demonstrate such a low level of competence in numeracy that this can lead to error and put patients at risk.

Problems with numeracy amongst the general population in the United Kingdom are well recognized and acknowledged as a cause of concern for successive govern-ments. Despite recurrent investment in projects supporting adult numeracy in the UK, up to half of the working population in England has been found to have mathematics skills that are no better than those expected of a primary school pupil (www.national-numeracy.org.uk, 2012). Since it is from this population that the majority of UK healthcare professionals are recruited, it is reasonable to conclude that numeracy skills may be inadequate within a significant proportion of the large workforce employed in the healthcare professions. This is now a recognized cause of concern for healthcare employers, educators and professional regulators.

Healthcare practitioners enter their chosen profession to improve people's lives and to perform their role safely, competently and to the best of their ability. All healthcare practitioners are educated to ensure they are competent in their roles and it is reassur-ing that most healthcare is delivered to patients safely and appropriately. However, inac-curate dose calculations by healthcare staff continue to occur, leading to medication errors. Drug dosage errors in the prescribing and administration of medications are a common cause of the patient safety incidents reported to the National Patient Safety Agency (NPSA) in the United Kingdom, and a leading cause of patient harm. In chil-dren, where the calculations can be more complex than in adults and where the patient's tolerance of error is lower, medication errors due to incorrect dosage or strength of medication continue to be significant and common causes of reported harm to patients. Calculation errors by a factor of 10, for example, are a common cause of such errors in paediatric settings.

All qualified healthcare practitioners have a duty to remain competent in their practice. Professional regulators such as the General Pharmaceutical Council, the Health Professions Council and the Nursing and Midwifery Council acknowledge the importance of numeracy skills in the role of their registrants. Each of these regulators sets minimum mathematics qualifications or standards of numeracy for entry to pre-registration educational programmes, progression within these programmes and final qualification. In writing this book we have ensured that the mathematical skills needed to meet such standards are covered in depth.

How is the book structured?

Although there are many books on the subject of numeracy we hope that this one will prove to be distinctive. First, it is structured around the mathematical ideas, drawing on healthcare contexts to illustrate and explain these. Second, rather than merely teaching rules for specific healthcare tasks, we aim to improve the reader's numeracy skills in a range of contexts through their understanding of mathematical concepts and principles and by building confidence in handling all kinds of numbers: whole numbers, decimals, fractions, percentages, and especially numbers in the context of measurement, such as dosages, rates and concentrations. Third, we do not assume that there is only one approved way of doing any particular kind of mathematical calculation, or that formal, written methods are superior to mental and informal strategies. We encourage the reader to be alert to how the relationships between numbers can be exploited and to use intuitive approaches to calculations. If after working through this book you still feel you need to use 'long multiplication' or a calculator to multiply 0.25 grams by 12, for example, then we have failed!

A set of specific numeracy objectives is set out at the start of each chapter. These objectives indicate what the practitioner should be able to do in a practical healthcare context when they have mastered the material in that chapter.

These objectives are followed by a feature called *Spot the errors* (except in Chapter 15). The reader is challenged to read quickly through a number of statements and to identify any mathematical errors. This section is intended to simulate the way that practitioners often have to deal with mathematical calculations and instructions under pressure without much time to stop and reflect. The errors are then identified and explained and, from Chapter 4 onwards, the significance of the errors in a healthcare context is discussed. If you spot all our deliberate errors, then you have our authority to give yourself a hearty pat on the back!

Each chapter then provides detailed explanation and illustration of the mathematical ideas and processes specified in the objectives, with examples of their application in practice and with key points highlighted in boxes throughout the text. At the end of each chapter there is a section called *Have a check-up*. This consists of some exercises for you to work through to check your learning of the content of that chapter; annotated answers to these check-up questions are given at the end of the book.

We have set out to write an accessible book on a subject that we know many readers find challenging. The book combines Derek's mathematical knowledge and understanding of the teaching and learning of the subject with Paul's clinical experience and understanding of the importance of numeracy in the healthcare environment. We hope that this combination will enable the reader to develop an understanding and confidence in the use of numbers in both their daily life and their professional practice.

How to use this book

The first thing to say is that to engage with the material in each chapter of this book you will need to work through the mathematics, with a pencil and paper; have a go at the *Spot the errors* section; work through the examples; do the check-up questions, don't just look up the answers! We recommend that you check our working and scribble your own mathematical jottings all over the book; this will help you to engage with the material (and help us by undermining the second-hand book market!).

For most readers we would recommend that you work through the book chapter by chapter. As we have explained above, the book is written to improve the reader's understanding of numeracy and their skills and confidence in using numbers. It takes the reader through the various mathematical processes and concepts, building their knowledge and understanding of these chapter by chapter. So it is best to work through the chapters in the order they are written, ensuring that you have a thorough understanding of the content of one chapter before moving on to the next. This approach will enable the gradual development of a broad understanding of the different processes and concepts that are likely to be encountered in healthcare practice and daily life. We hope that you will then want to use the book in the future as a reference book, to revise and reinforce particular skills and to check up on things you have forgotten.

A DISCLAIMER

Readers should be aware that the healthcare examples used in this book are chosen to illustrate and explain specific mathematical ideas. While we have taken care to make these examples as genuine as possible and to use realistic or recommended doses of particular drugs, it must be understood that this book is not a manual for healthcare practice or a guide to drug dosages.

UNDERSTANDING THE NUMBER SYSTEM

1

OBJECTIVES

The practitioner should be able to:

- understand the place-value principle in our number system for both whole numbers and decimal numbers
- use and interpret powers of 10
- recognize the positions of whole numbers or decimal numbers on a section of a number line
- appreciate where zeros are needed in decimal numbers
- express a decimal number as tenths, hundredths or thousandths

Our mission throughout this book is to increase your understanding of mathematics, because we know that this will help to make you a more confident and competent health-care practitioner. So, we begin with refreshing your understanding of numbers! The purpose of this chapter is to remind you of some fundamental ideas about whole numbers and decimals and to ensure that you have a clearer grasp of how our base-ten place-value number system works. The practitioner will need to be able to apply this understanding of the number system in the context of their healthcare practice, especially when the numbers are used in measurement. Various aspects of measurement are not explained until Chapters 4–7 of this book, so it is from those chapters on that we will illustrate and apply mathematical ideas more specifically in healthcare contexts.

SPOT THE ERRORS

Identify any obvious mathematical errors in the following ten statements.

1 The digit 7 in the number 87 654 represents seven thousand.

2 Counting in ones, the next number after three thousand and ninety-nine is four thousand.

3 On a number line 8050 lies halfway between 8000 and 8100.

4 To calculate the cost per day of a 28-day course of medicine costing £75.60, a pharmacist enters 75.60 ÷ 28 on a calculator and gets the result 2.7; this means the cost per day is two pounds and seven pence.

5 The number 0.0008 is 'eight ten-thousandths'.

6 The number halfway between 0.007 and 0.008 is 0.075.

7 The number 4567 is equal to $(4 \times 10^3) + (5 \times 10^2) + (6 \times 10^1) + (7 \times 10^0)$.

8 The number 0.067 is equal to $(6 \times 10^{-2}) + (7 \times 10^{-3})$.

9 In this set {0.09, 0.8, 0.084, 0.18, 0.48}, the greatest number is 0.8 and the smallest number is 0.084.

10 1.275 is equal to 1 unit and 275 thousandths, which is 1275 thousandths.

(errors identified on page 4)

How does place value work?

Over history there have been many systems for representing numbers. The system used internationally today is essentially a Hindu-Arabic system that has ten as its base and uses the principle of *place value*. This principle means that, for example, the symbol '5' occurring in a numeral might sometimes mean 'five' (as in 65), but it could mean 'fifty' (as in 56) or 'five thousand', as in (5678), or 'five hundredths' (as in 2.75), and so on, depending on the *place* in which it is written. Most ancient number systems did not use this principle. For example, in Roman numerals the symbol 'V' wherever it is written, for example in XV or in CLXVIII, means 'five'.

Numeral and number

A numeral is a symbol used to represent a number. For example, the number of teeth that an adult should have is represented by the numeral 32.

The place-value system for numbers is based on *powers* of ten. These are: one, ten, a hundred, a thousand, ten thousand, a hundred thousand, a million, and so on, getting ten times bigger each time. These powers of ten can be expressed symbolically and in words in a number of ways as shown in the table in Figure 1.1.

one	1	10^0	ten to the power 0	1
ten	10	10^1	ten to the power 1	1 × 10
a hundred	100	10^2	ten to the power 2	1 × 10 × 10
a thousand	1000	10^3	ten to the power 3	1 × 10 × 10 × 10
ten thousand	10 000	10^4	ten to the power 4	1 × 10 × 10 × 10 × 10
a hundred thousand	100 000	10^5	ten to the power 5	1 × 10 × 10 × 10 × 10 × 10
a million	1 000 000	10^6	ten to the power 6	1 × 10 × 10 × 10 × 10 × 10 × 10

Figure 1.1   A table showing increasing powers of 10

There are a few things to note here. In general, ten to the power n (10^n) means 1 multiplied by 10, n times, and this is equal to a number written as 1 followed by n zeros. For example, 10^9 would be 1 multiplied by 9 tens: $1 \times 10 \times 10 \times 10 \times 10 \times 10 \times 10 \times 10 \times 10 \times 10$; written out in full as a numeral this number (a billion) is 1 followed by 9 zeros.

The expression 10^2 (ten to the power 2) is also read as 'ten squared'; and 10^3 (ten to the power 3) is also read as 'ten cubed'.

We have included 'ten to the power zero' at the top of the table above, as a way of writing the number 1. Although this might seem a bit weird, you should at least be able to see how it fits into the pattern of the table. This use of 'to the power zero' is a mathematical convention adopted for the sake of completeness; it also provides a bridge for extending the place-value system from whole numbers to decimal numbers (see below). Think of it as meaning '1 not multiplied by any tens' or '1 followed by no zeros'.

This table could go on for ever, continuing with ten million, a hundred million, a billion, ten billion, and so on. But the larger the power of ten the less useful becomes the actual name. For example, 'a trillion' might not convey much to us, until someone tells

ERRORS IDENTIFIED

The obvious errors are in Statements 2, 4 and 6.

Statement 2

The next number after three thousand and ninety-nine (3099) is three thousand one hundred (3100). We hope this is obvious now you see the numbers written as numerals.

Statement 4

The cost is two pounds and seventy pence (£2.70) per day. The numbers 2.7, 2.70, 2.700, 2.7000, and so on, all represent the same quantity, since the zeros simply tell us that there are no tenths, no hundredths, no thousandths, and so on. Calculators usually do not display these 'trailing zeros' and will give any of these results as 2.7. The '7' in this context means '7 tenths of a pound', which is seven ten-pences, or seventy pence. For sums of money the convention (which calculators ignore) is always to write them with two digits after the point, in order to avoid this kind of confusion.

Statement 6

The number halfway between 0.007 and 0.008 is actually 0.0075. This is more obvious if we write all the numbers with four digits after the decimal point: 0.0070, 0.0075, 0.0080. They are shown on a number-line diagram in Figure 1.2, along with a few other numbers in their vicinity.

(now continue reading from page 3)

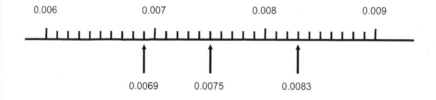

Figure 1.2   A number-line diagram from 0.006 to 0.009

us that it actually stands for 10^{12} (1 followed by 12 zeros). An important (and very large) number in science that we will mention in Chapter 14 involves 10^{23}; written like this, as a power of ten, this is much easier to grasp than referring to it as 'a hundred sextillion'!

Note also that we use the recognized convention for writing numbers with more than four digits: the digits are grouped in threes from the right, and then written with spaces between the groups of three. So, a million is correctly written 1 000 000, not 1,000,000. The reason for this is that some countries use a comma where we use a decimal point.

Having got these powers of ten, we can now see how our base-ten place-value number system works. First, we need only ten digits: 0, 1, 2, 3, 4, 5, 6, 7, 8, 9, and with these we can (theoretically) count any number in the universe! We count beyond 9 by using the place-value principle: the value of a digit in a numeral depends on where it is written. As we work from right to left (for whole numbers) the first place we might write a digit represents 'ones' (sometimes called units), the next place 'tens', the next 'hundreds', the next 'thousands', and so on. So, the numeral, 2345, for example, represents '5 ones, 4 tens, 3 hundreds and 2 thousands'.

Digits

A *digit* is one of the ten symbols used to construct numerals: 0, 1, 2, 3, 4, 5, 6, 7, 8 and 9.

But, of course, we actually read these numbers from left to right – and we use certain language conventions when expressing the numbers in words. So we read 2345 as: 'two thousand, three hundred and forty-five'. 'Forty' here is shorthand for 'four tens', of course.

This system means that the digit at the front of the number (on the left) is the most significant, because it always represents the greatest quantity – and the digits become less significant in terms of what they represent as we move to the right. We discuss the idea of 'significant digits' further in Chapter 8.

So, the numeral 2345 is a condensed way of representing a number that could also be written in full as: $2000 + 300 + 40 + 5$.

Or, using powers of ten: $(2 \times 10^3) + (3 \times 10^2) + (4 \times 10^1) + (5 \times 10^0)$.

EXAMPLE 1.1

What are the values represented by the digits 3 and 0 in 53 028? How do you read this number out loud? What is it expressed in powers of 10?

(a) The digit 3 represents 3 thousands, or 3000, or 3×10^3.

The digit 0 (zero) represents 'no hundreds', or 0×10^2.

(b) This number is read as: 'fifty-three thousand and twenty-eight'.

(c) $53\ 028 = (5 \times 10^4) + (3 \times 10^3) + (0 \times 10^2) + (2 \times 10^1) + (8 \times 10^0)$.

The digit zero in a numeral like 53 028 is called a 'place-holder', occupying an otherwise empty place (there are no hundreds) and ensuring that the preceding digits are in their correct place. In the history of our number system the invention of a symbol for zero for this purpose was a highly significant breakthrough. This aspect of zero is particularly important in some decimal numbers, as we shall see below.

How are numbers positioned on a number line or numerical scale?

Number lines, particularly in the form of various measuring scales, are important in healthcare practice. They are all derived from the simple idea of representing numbers as points on a line. This enables us to recognize visually the positional relationship between numbers. We start with simple number lines using only whole numbers.

Figure 1.3(a) shows a section of a number line from 2000 to 5000. Each step on this line represents a thousand, as we progress from 2000 to 3000, to 4000, to 5000. The number 3758 must lie on this line, somewhere between 3000 and 4000, because it is greater than 3000 and less than 4000. In Figure 1.3(b) the section between 3000 and 4000 is shown enlarged and divided into ten equal sections. Each of these sections must represent a step of a hundred along the line (because ten hundreds equal a thousand). So the points marked on the number line in (b) are 3000, 3100, 3200, 3300, and so on,

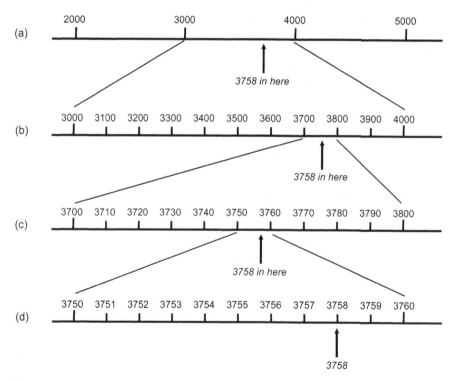

Figure 1.3   Locating 3758 on a number line

up to 4000. The number we are chasing lies between 3700 and 3800. So, in Figure 1.3(c) we have expanded this section of the line and again divided it up into ten equal sections. Each of these sections now represents a step of 10 along the line (because ten 10s equal a hundred). So the points marked on the line in (c) are 3700, 3710, 3720, 3730, and so on, up to 3800. Our number (3758) now lies between 3750 and 3760. So we repeat the process in 1.3(d), where the ten equal sections between 3750 and 3760 are now steps of one: 3750, 3751, 3752, and so on. Now we can see exactly where 3758 lies.

OK, so we have rather laboured the point here! But this way of seeing numbers is absolutely crucial in reading scales, as well as in having a sense of how numbers relate to each other in terms of order and relative position. And this process of repeatedly subdividing spaces between consecutive numbers on a scale into ten equal sections will be particularly important in your understanding of decimal numbers.

So, how does place value work with decimal numbers?

The building blocks of decimal numbers

A tenth = 0.1
A hundredth = 0.01
A thousandth = 0.001

Just as we can divide thousands into ten hundreds, hundreds into ten tens, and tens into ten ones, we can continue dividing sections of the number line repeatedly into ten smaller parts, generating tenths, hundredths, thousandths, and so on. A tenth is what you get if you divide a unit into ten equal parts. A hundredth is what you get if you divide a tenth into ten equal parts. A thousandth is what you get if you divide a hundredth into ten equal parts. And so on.

So this is how we are able to represent quantities less than 1, using decimal numbers. We put a 'decimal point' (a full stop) after the digit representing ones (units), and then continue with digits representing these smaller quantities. So, the 1 in the decimal number 0.1 means a tenth; in 0.01 it means a hundredth; in 0.001 it means a thousandth, and so on. These are the building blocks of decimal numbers.

Then, for example, in the decimal number 2.358, the 2 represents 2 ones (2 units); the 3 represents 3 tenths of a unit; the 5 represents 5 hundredths of a unit; and the 8 represents 8 thousandths of a unit.

Surprisingly, tenths, hundredths, thousandths, ten thousandths, and so on, can also be expressed as powers of ten. This is done by following the patterns in the table in Figure 1.4, continuing the powers of ten from zero into negative numbers: 0, –1, –2, –3, and so on. There's no need to be puzzled by these negative powers of ten: just accept the notation as a convenient (and actually rather clever) mathematical convention for representing the smaller and smaller subdivisions into ten equal parts.

Figure 1.4 is a table showing tenths, hundredths, and so on, how they are written as decimal numbers, and the corresponding negative powers of ten.

Again, there are a few things to note. First, just be aware of how this table is generated by continuing a pattern to produce smaller and smaller quantities, each a tenth of the preceding one, and how these can be expressed using the variety of language and notation. So, for example, 'a thousandth' is written as the decimal numeral 0.001; as a power

Negative powers of 10

An example:
$$10^{-4} = 0.0001$$
$$= 1 \div 10 \div 10 \div 10 \div 10$$

one	1	10^0	ten to the power 0	1
a tenth	0.1	10^{-1}	ten to the power −1	1 ÷ 10
a hundredth	0.01	10^{-2}	ten to the power −2	1 ÷ 10 ÷ 10
a thousandth	0.001	10^{-3}	ten to the power −3	1 ÷ 10 ÷ 10 ÷ 10
a ten thousandth	0.0001	10^{-4}	ten to the power −4	1 ÷ 10 ÷ 10 ÷ 10 ÷ 10
a hundred thousandth	0.000 01	10^{-5}	ten to the power −5	1 ÷ 10 ÷ 10 ÷ 10 ÷ 10 ÷ 10
a millionth	0.000 001	10^{-6}	ten to the power −6	1 ÷ 10 ÷ 10 ÷ 10 ÷ 10 ÷ 10 ÷ 10

Figure 1.4 A table showing decreasing powers of 10 below zero

of 10 it is 10^{-3} (ten to the power negative 3); it is also what you get if you *divide* 1 by 10 three times (1 ÷ 10 ÷ 10 ÷ 10). To see this pattern in action, enter 1 onto a calculator then divide by 10 repeatedly. This helps us to interpret a negative power of 10, like 10^{-3}. It just means divide one by ten, 3 times!

Note also that the same convention applies for grouping digits after the decimal point in threes as applies for the digits in front of the decimal point.

Note further that we have written a zero in front of the decimal point in each of the numbers 0.1, 0.01, 0.001, and so on. This addition of a leading zero is not strictly necessary; it is there just to make sure we spot the decimal point! This is particularly important in healthcare practice, where a dose written, say, as .5 grams might be misread as 5 grams. The zeros after the decimal point in 0.01 and 0.001 are necessary place-holders, of course. (Grams and other units of weight are explained in Chapter 6.)

Then, of course, this table could continue for ever, producing smaller and smaller quantities, each one of them a tenth of the previous one. So, for example, one molecule of common salt (sodium chloride) would weigh about 10^{-22} grams. This means taking a gram and dividing it into 10 parts, dividing one of these into 10 parts, dividing one of these into 10 parts, and continuing to do this 22 times in total.

We now have all we need to represent numbers that have parts smaller than 1 – what are called decimal numbers. Consider, for example, the decimal numeral 3.758. This is read as 'three point seven five eight'. It stands for 3 ones (units), 7 tenths, 5 hundredths and 8 thousandths. This can also be written in expanded form as: 3 + 0.7 + 0.05 + 0.008.

Or, using powers of ten: $(3 \times 10^0) + (7 \times 10^{-1}) + (5 \times 10^{-2}) + (8 \times 10^{-3})$.

EXAMPLE 1.2

What are the values represented by the digits 3 and 2 in 5.3028? How do you read this number out loud? What is it expressed in powers of 10?

(a) The digit 3 represents 3 tenths, or 0.3, or 3×10^{-1}.

The digit 2 represents 2 thousandths, 0.002, or 2×10^{-3}.

(b) This number is read as: 'five point three zero two eight'.

(c) $5.3028 = (5 \times 10^{0}) + (3 \times 10^{-1}) + (0 \times 10^{-2}) + (2 \times 10^{-3}) + (8 \times 10^{-4})$.

Figure 1.5 shows how we can locate the number 3.758 on the number line. Notice that Figure 1.5 is identical to Figure 1.3 (apart from the labels). This shows that place value works in exactly the same way beyond the decimal point as it does before it.

So, in Figure 1.5(a) 3.758 lies somewhere between 3 and 4, because the first digit tells us that we have three units and the '.758' tells us we have some other bits of a unit to add to this. So, we follow the process we used in Figure 1.3: divide the section from 3 to 4 into ten equal steps, each of which is a tenth of a unit, giving us 3, 3.1, 3.2, 3.3, and so on. Our number (3.758) lies between 3.7 and 3.8, as shown in Figure 1.5(b). In (c) the section from 3.7 to 3.8 is divided into ten equal steps, this time using hundredths of a unit, giving us 3.7, 3.71, 3.72, 3.73, and so on. Our number (3.758) lies between 3.75 and 3.76. In (d) we divide this into ten equal steps (thousandths), and hence we locate 3.758. As we move from (a) to (d) in Figure 1.5, we can see that our number 3.758 is (a) 3 units + (b) 7 tenths + (c) 5 hundredths + (d) 8 thousandths.

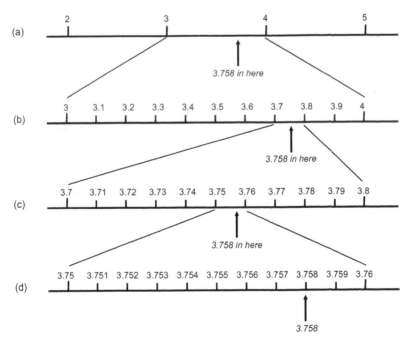

Figure 1.5 Locating 3.758 on a number line

EXAMPLE 1.3

On the section of a number line shown in Figure 1.6, (approximately) what are the numbers indicated by A, B and C?

The steps from 0.3 to 0.4, from 0.4 to 0.5, and so on, are steps of a tenth of a unit (0.1). These are then divided into 10 equal parts by the smaller gradations on the line, which therefore give steps of a hundredth (0.01). The points marked from 0.3 to 0.4, for example, are 0.3, 0.31, 0.32, 0.33, ... 0.39, 0.4.

So, A is 0.32 and, similarly, B is 0.45. Note that B is the midpoint between 0.4 and 0.5.

C is about halfway between 0.56 and 0.57, so, imagining the gap between 0.56 and 0.57 divided into ten (even smaller) sections (thousandths), C would be at about 0.565. C represents 5 tenths, 6 hundredths and 5 thousandths.

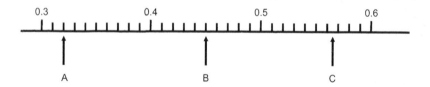

Figure 1.6   Number line section for Example 1.3

What else is there to know about zeros in decimal numbers?

In Figure 1.6, it is probably easier to identify the points A and B if we write the points on the scale as 0.30, 0.40, 0.50 and 0.60. Sticking a zero on the ends of these decimals doesn't change their values at all, because the zeros mean simply 'and no hundredths'. The points marked from 0.3 onwards (including 0.3) are then 0.30, 0.31, 0.32, 0.33, 0.34, 0.35, 0.36, 0.37, 0.38, 0.39, 0.40. Now this looks very similar to counting from 30 to 40! Notice also that it is much more obvious that B, being half-way between 0.40 and 0.50, must be 0.45. In the same way, in identifying C, if we think of 0.56 and 0.57 as 0.560 and 0.570, it is much easier to see that the point in the middle between them is 0.565. Have a look again at the correction to *Spot the errors* Statement 6 at the beginning of this chapter. The zeros we are exploiting here are called *trailing zeros*.

Zeros in numerals have some important roles to play! We have earlier commented on the role of zero in our number system as a place-holder, in numbers like 5007 (no hundreds, no tens) or 5.007 (no tenths, no hundredths). We have also noted the convention of placing an additional leading zero in front of a decimal point if there are no other digits there. Technically, we could place as many zeros as we wish at the front of a number – for example, 2.56 = 02.56 = 002.56 = 0002.56, and so on – because these zeros simply tell us that there are no tens no hundreds, no thousands, and so on – although it is not often that we would have a reason to do this. Occasionally it helps in doing some calculations, to ensure that we have all the ones, tens and hundreds, and so on, lined up correctly. Another area where we often use leading zeros is in recording time. At the time of writing this sentence it is 09:05 on 08.05.2012. Here we are using the convention of putting a leading zero in front of a single digit to give the hour, the number of minutes, the day and the month all with two digits – probably reflecting digital displays of dates and times.

But you will find that trailing zeros are quite often used in decimal numbers. A decimal number, such as 2.75, could also be written as 2.750, 2.7500, 2.75000, and so on, with as many of these trailing zeros as we wish. Trailing zeros like these are used particularly to ensure that that a group of numbers or measurements are all being given to the same level of accuracy. For example in a men's 100-metres race the times would be recorded in hundredths of a second, so they would appear with two digits after the decimal point. If one runner's time is 9.9 seconds, this would be given as 9.90, so that it can be more easily compared with the other times of 9.92, 9.89, 9.85 and 9.96 seconds. We have seen in Example 1.3 above how handy it is sometimes to stick one or two additional trailing zeros on decimal numbers.

Note that calculators do not show trailing zeros in the results of calculations. If you use a calculator to add £1.26 and £3.44, for example, the result displayed will be 4.7, which you then have to interpret as £4.70. (See *Spot the error* Statement 4 and its correction.)

EXAMPLE 1.4

(a) Put these numbers in order, from the smallest to the greatest: 0.9, 0.091, 0.91, 0.019, 0.19, 0.09.

Add trailing zeros so that all the numbers have three digits after the decimal points: 0.900, 0.091, 0.910, 0.019, 0.190, 0.090.

Now it is easier to put them in order: 0.019, 0.090, 0.091, 0.190, 0.900, 0.910.

Now dropping the trailing zeros, they are in order: 0.019, 0.09, 0.091, 0.19, 0.9, 0.91.

(b) What time comes halfway between 33.8 seconds and 33.9 seconds?

Add a trailing zero to each time so they become: 33.80 and 33.90 seconds. It is now clear that halfway between them is 33.85 seconds.

How do you read and interpret decimal numbers?

Although we might say 'two pounds ninety' when reading £2.90 – because we see the 90 as representing 90 pence – it is not correct to read the decimal number 2.90 as 'two point ninety'. It should be read as 'two point nine zero'. Similarly, 5.67 is not 'five point sixty-seven' is it 'five point six seven'. The reason for this is that if you say 'five point sixty-seven' the response could be 'sixty-seven what?'

The actual answer to that question is 'sixty-seven hundredths'. When you see 5.67, the 6 means 6 tenths and the 7 means 7 hundredths. But, because a tenth is ten hundredths, the 6 tenths are equivalent to 60 hundredths. So, together with the 7 hundredths, the digits after the decimal point are equivalent to 67 hundredths in total. So, 5.67 (read as five point six seven) is equal to 5 units and 67 hundredths. Furthermore, since the 5 units are equivalent to 500 hundredths of a unit, the whole 5.67 is equal to 567 hundredths. That's just like saying £5.67 is equal to 567 pence.

Here's another example: 1.025 (one point zero two five). How can we interpret this? Well, as it stands it means 1 unit, 2 hundredths and 5 thousandths. But the 2 hundredths are equivalent to 20 thousandths, so 1.025 can be seen as 1 unit and 25 thousandths. Then, because the 1 unit is equivalent to 1000 thousandths, we could convert the entire number to 1025 thousandths. So, 1.025 = 1025 thousandths.

This way of looking at decimal numbers is very important when it comes to converting measurements between different units, as we shall see in Chapters 4 to 6. In Chapter 4, for example, we will see how a measurement of 1.75 metres is converted to 175 centimetres (hundredths of a metre). And, in Chapter 5, how 1.750 litres is converted to 1750 millilitres (thousandths of a litre).

EXAMPLE 1.5

(a) Write in tenths: 12.5

12.5 = 12 units and 5 tenths = 125 tenths

(b) Write in hundredths: 2.25; 12.33; 0.8

2.25 = 2 units and 25 hundredths = 225 hundredths

12.33 = 12 units and 33 hundredths = 1233 hundredths

0.8 = 0.80 = 80 hundredths.

(c) Write in thousandths: 0.175; 0.067; 5.67

0.175 = 0 units and 175 thousandths = 175 thousandths

0.067 = 0 units and 67 thousandths = 67 thousandths

5.67 = 5.670 = 5 units and 670 thousandths = 5670 thousandths.

1.1   Consider the numeral 72 405.

(a) In words, what does the 2 represent?
(b) Write your answer to part (a) using a power of 10.
(c) What does the zero represent?

1.2   In the decimal numeral 0.9208,

(a) in words, what does the 2 represent?
(b) Write your answer to part (a) using a power of 10;
(c) what does the zero after the 2 represent?

1.3   Which is the largest and which the smallest in this list of numbers:

5.601, 5.61, 5.061, 5.16, 5.016, 5.106?

1.4   Which number lies halfway between:

(a) 0.08 and 0.09?
(b) 0.1 and 0.11?

1.5   (a) Which is the larger: 1×10^7 or a million?
(b) Which is the smaller: 1×10^{-7} or a millionth?

1.6   In Figure 1.2 the main points on the scale are labelled 0.006, 0.007, 0.008, 0.009.

(a) How would the next main point in this sequence be marked?
(b) Roughly, where would the point labelled 100 be on this scale?

1.7   Identify (approximately) the numbers labelled A, B and C in Figure 1.7.

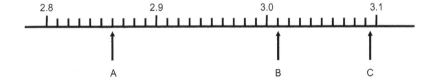

Figure 1.7   Number line section for check-up question 1.7

1.8   The labels on the section of the number line shown in Figure 1.8 have been removed. But the arrows indicate where on this line 0.301 and 0.309 would come. What are the labels missing from the four boxes?

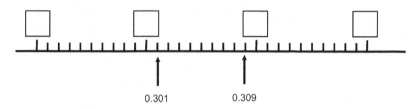

0.301   0.309

Figure 1.8   Number line section for check-up question 1.8

1.9   (See Example 1.5.) Write:
      (a) 0.275 as thousandths;
      (b) 25.6 as tenths;
      (c) 12.5 as hundredths;
      (d) 1.05 as thousandths.

ADDITION AND SUBTRACTION SKILLS

2

OBJECTIVES

The practitioner should be able to:

- use their knowledge of addition and subtraction facts to add or subtract multiples of 10, 100 or 1000
- draw on a range of informal strategies for addition and subtraction, both mental and written, appropriate to the numbers involved
- use empty number line diagrams to support mental calculations
- apply accurately a column method for addition involving whole numbers with any number of digits
- make sensible decisions about when to do addition and subtraction calculations by informal methods, by formal methods or by using a calculator

---

In this chapter we aim to encourage you to develop your mental and informal written methods of doing addition and subtraction, making use of whatever number facts you know and with which you are confident. A lot of what we do here is just to make explicit the kinds of mental strategies that most numerate people employ as a matter of course. In the busy life of a healthcare practitioner there's a lot to be said for having access to a range of calculation strategies that you can call on with confidence – and, of course, accuracy!

Note that this chapter is about calculations with whole numbers. Calculations involving decimal numbers are explained in Chapter 9. A few of our examples in this chapter involve millilitres, which are units of liquid volume explained in Chapter 5.

In deciding what to cover here, we have assumed that the reader has some basic knowledge of number facts. For example, we assume that you can at least: (a) recall instantly additions of single-digit numbers, such as 3 + 7 and 8 + 9; (b) recall instantly subtractions from a number up to 20, such as 13 – 5 and 20 – 17; (c) do instantly an addition or subtraction involving a multiple of 10 and a single-digit number, such as 230 + 7 and 70 – 8. If you are at all hesitant about this level of calculation, then, if you want to be a numerate healthcare practitioner, write out loads of examples for yourself and practise!

SPOT THE ERRORS

Identify any obvious errors in the calculations in the following ten statements. Do not use a calculator. You should not need to use a formal written method for calculations like these.

1 56 + 57 = 113

2 256 + 137 = (200 + 50 + 6) + (100 + 30 + 7) = 300 + 80 + 13 = 393

3 267 + 198 = 267 + 200 – 2 = 467 – 2 = 465

4 53 tablets from a packet of 120 have been used, so 77 remain.

5 1003 – 929 = 126

6 300 – 148 = 300 – 150 + 2 = 150 + 2 = 152.

7 1000 – 899 = 1001 – 900 = 101

8 250 – 63 can be found by adding on from 63: add 7 (to get to 70), add 30 (to get to 100), add 100 (to get to 200) + 50 (to get to 250) = 7 + 30 + 100 + 50 = 187.

9 A patient has a total fluid intake from midnight up to 7 am recorded as 648 millilitres; in the next hour the patient receives an intravenous infusion of 83 millilitres and drinks 150 millilitres. So the total fluid intake up to 8 am is 648 + 83 + 150 = 881 millilitres.

10 A patient with fluid intake of 2718 millilitres and a fluid output of 2035 millilitres in one day has a positive fluid balance of 683 millilitres, because 2718 – 2035 = 683.

(errors identified on page 18)

How is knowledge of addition and subtraction facts used to add or subtract multiples of 10, 100 or 1000?

A *multiple* of 10 is what you get if you multiply 10 by some whole number. So all these numbers are multiples of 10: 20 (2 tens), 70 (7 tens), 120 (12 tens), 200 (20 tens), and so on; in other words, any whole number ending in zero.

Similarly, all these are multiples of 100: 200, 700, 1200, 2000, and so on; any whole number ending in two zeros. And these are examples of multiples of 1000: 2000, 7000, 12 000, 20 000; any whole number ending in three zeros.

So, the first thing we want you to realize is that if you know, say, that 5 + 9 = 14, then you also know that 50 + 90 = 140 (5 tens + 9 tens = 14 tens). And you also know 500 + 900 = 1400 (5 hundreds + 9 hundreds = 14 hundreds) and 5000 + 9000 = 14 000 (5 thousands + 9 thousands = 14 thousands).

The same principles apply to subtraction, of course. So, if you know, that 20 – 7 = 13, then you also know these results: 200 – 70 = 130; 2000 – 700 = 1300; and 20 000 – 7000 = 13 000.

Multiples

Multiples of 10 are: 10, 20, 30, 40, 50, 60, 70, 80, 90, 100, 110, 120, 130, ...

Multiples of 100 are: 100, 200, 300, 400, 500, 600, 700, 800, 900, 1000, 1100, ...

Multiples of 1000 are: 1000, 2000, 3000, 4000, 5000, ...

If you know ...

27 + 4 = 31
then you also know:
270 + 40 = 310
2700 + 400 = 3100
27 000 + 4000 = 31 000
and so on.

EXAMPLE 2.1

(a) 12 000 women and 9000 men are on a national training programme. How many is that altogether?

The calculation required is 12 000 + 9000. Both numbers are multiples of 1000, so, knowing 12 + 9 = 21, we can write down 12 000 + 9000 = 21 000.

(b) 700 millilitres of an infusion containing a total of 1500 millilitres have been delivered. How many millilitres remain? (Millilitres as units of liquid volume are explained in Chapter 5.)

The calculation required is 1500 – 700. Both numbers are multiples of 100, so, knowing 15 – 7, we can write down 1500 – 700 = 800. So, 800 millilitres remain.

ERRORS IDENTIFIED

The obvious errors are in Statements 4 and 5.

Statement 4

The correct answer is that 67 remain, because 120 – 53 = 67.

Statement 5

The correct answer is 1003 – 929 = 74.

These are two examples of common errors that are made in subtraction calculations with one or more zeros in the first number. They are typical of the kinds of errors that practitioners can make when working under pressure. So remember to raise a red alert signal in your brain when you see a zero in a subtraction! We suggest methods below to avoid errors like these.

(now continue reading from page 17)

How can additions and subtractions be done mentally and informally?

Mental strategies for + and -

Look carefully at the numbers involved and see if any of these strategies might be useful:

1 Stepping-stones
2 Empty number-line diagrams
3 Partitioning into 100s, 10s and 1s
4 Bridging the gap
5 Using an equivalent subtraction
6 Compensation
7 Starting with friendlier numbers

We offer below a number of strategies that can be drawn on to support mental calculations. Having these kind of informal ways of manipulating the numbers involved in an addition or a subtraction gives a person greater confidence in numerical situations and is a key component of numeracy.

Strategy 1: Use multiples of 10 or 100 as stepping-stones in addition

This strategy is based on knowing what you add to make a number up to the next multiple of 10 or 100. For example, if you have to find 37 + 8, you may well think along these lines: I need 3 to get from 37 to 40, so split the 8 into 3 + 5 … so that's 37 + 3 + 5, which is 40 + 5 = 45. We like to think that what we are doing is using 40 (the next multiple of 10 after 37) as a *stepping-stone* to the result, 45. Of course, you don't need to write any of this down; we are just trying to represent your mental reasoning. We hope that all we are doing is making explicit what you do intuitively anyway!

EXAMPLE 2.2

(a) Find 198 + 7. Use 200 as a stepping-stone. We need 2 to make the 198 up to 200.

Think of the 7 as 2 + 5; then 198 + 7 = 198 + 2 + 5 = 200 + 5 = 205.

(b) Find 995 + 18. Use 1000 as a stepping-stone. We need 5 to make the 995 up to 1000.

Think of the 18 as 5 + 13; then 995 + 18 = 995 + 5 + 13 = 1000 + 13 = 1013.

Strategy 2: Use empty number lines to support your mental reasoning

An empty number line is a number line without a scale on it. So, it's just a line! But then we jot numbers on this line, not worrying about any scale or accuracy in where we position them, as long as they are in the right order.

Figure 2.1 shows how we used (a) 200 and (b) 1000 as stepping-stones in Example 2.2. In (a) to add 7 to 198 we do it in two steps of 2 and 5, stepping on 200 on the way to the result, 205. Similarly, in (b) to add 18 to 995 we do it in two steps of 5 and 13, stepping on 1000 on our way to the result, 1013.

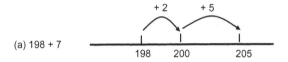

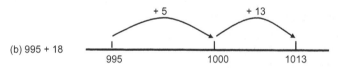

Figure 2.1   Empty number lines for Example 2.2, using (a) 200 and (b) 1000 as stepping-stones

The empty number line picture is particularly useful in supporting our mental reason-ing in doing subtraction calculations, as we shall explain below in connection with some other strategies. Consider, for example, 1005 – 17. When you are subtracting a relatively small number like this it is often effective to imagine working back along a number line. Figure 2.2 illustrates how we could this in this example, imaging the 17 as a step of 10, followed by a step of 5 and finally a step of 2.

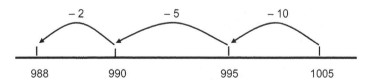

Figure 2.2   Calculating 1005 – 17

In doing additions it is often best to start with the larger number. For example, if in Example 2.2 we had been given (a) 7 + 198 and (b) 18 + 995, it would be quite hard to think of (a) starting at 7 and then counting on by 198, or (b) starting at 18 and counting on by 995! So, as a general rule, it is often easier to switch round additions like these, so we imagine that we have the larger number and we are adding to it the smaller number.

Strategy 3: For additions, mentally partition numbers into thousands, hundreds, tens and ones (units)

Say, for example, we have to find 17 + 76. First, we switch the order and think of it as 76 + 17. Then we expect that you would think of the 17 as 10 + 7. Adding the 10 is easy, so we now have 86 + 7, which (using strategy 1) is 93.

Partitioning a number means imagining it (or, if necessary, writing it down) in expanded form, in thousands, hundreds, tens and ones (units) – as we did in Chapter 1 when explaining place value. So, for example, given 376 we would think of it as '300 + 70 + 6'. Given 293 we would think '200 + 90 + 3'.

So, to find 376 + 293, we might think (300 + 70 + 6) + (200 + 90 + 3).

We then add the hundreds: 300 + 200 = 500. Then add the tens: 70 + 90 = 160. Finally add the units, 6 + 3 = 9. So 376 + 293 becomes 500 + 160 + 9, which equals 660 + 9 = 669. This looks long-winded written out, but you should be able to do this process mentally in a couple of seconds, maybe with just one or two jottings to help you remember where you are.

Note that in doing mental additions like this we use a *front-end* approach. This means that we begin with the digits at the front of the numbers, the ones that have the greatest place value, and work from left to right. Intuitively this makes most sense, but notice that this contrasts with formal written methods for addition, in which we usually start with the units and work from right to left.

Below are some more examples, showing the mental processes we might use for various additions. Note that sometimes we partition both numbers. Other times we might need to partition just one of them.

EXAMPLE 2.3

(a) 375 + 275 = (300 + 70 + 5) + (200 + 70 + 5) = (300 + 200) + (70 + 70) + (5 + 5) = 500 + 140 + 10 = 650.

(b) 18 + 63 = 63 + 18 = 63 + (10 + 8) = 73 + 8 = 81.

(c) 127 + 68 = (100 + 20 + 7) + (60 + 8) = 100 + (20 + 60) + (7 + 8) = 100 + 80 + 15 = 195.

(d) 4750 + 3200 = 4750 + (3000 + 200) = 7750 + 200 = 7950.

Strategy 4: Think of subtraction as bridging the gap

A subtraction like 275 – 87 does not just mean, 'Take 87 away from 275, what is left?' It might also mean: (1) what is the difference between 275 and 87? (2) how many (or much) more is 275 than 87? (3) how many (or much) fewer (or less) than 275 is 87? (4) what do you add to 87 to get 275?

These different ways of interpreting subtraction suggest some important and useful strategies for doing actual calculations, like 275 – 87. In each of questions (1), (2) and (3) above we could imagine 275 and 87 positioned on a number line and then having to find the size of the gap between them (see Figure 2.3(a)). So how do we find the size of the gap? There may be a number of ways of doing this, but in question (4) we get the clue that one way is to start at the 87 and add on numbers until we get to the 275. Figure 2.3(b) shows how this might be done. Starting at 87, add 3 to get to 90; add 10 to get to 100; add 100 to get to 200; add 75 to get to 275. So the gap is equal to 3 + 10 + 100 + 75 = 188. You may well choose to bridge the gap in different ways, maybe using more steps or fewer steps.

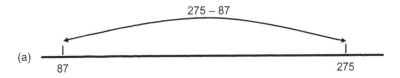

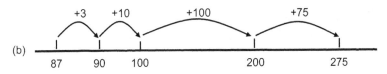

Figure 2.3   Finding 275 – 87 by bridging the gap between 87 and 275

EXAMPLE 2.4

How much fluid would bring a patient's total fluid intake in a 12-hour period up from 465 millilitres to 1200 millilitres? (For millilitres, see Chapter 5.)

Imagine 465 and 1200 on a number line. We can bridge the gap by adding on from 465: add 5, to get to 470; add 30 to get to 500; add 700 to get to 1200. Altogether we have to add 5 + 30 + 700 = 735.

So 735 millilitres is the volume of fluid required. The calculation we have done here by a series of simple additions is 1200 – 465.

This approach is particularly easy with the subtraction questions that cause the most difficulties when using formal methods: those with zeros in the first number, like the 1200 – 465 in Example 2.4 above; and also like the incorrect Statements 4 and 5 in *Spot the errors* at the start of the chapter. Figure 2.4 shows clearly why the correct answers to these are: (a) 120 – 53 = 7 + 60 = 67; and (b) 1003 – 929 = 1 + 70 + 3 = 74.

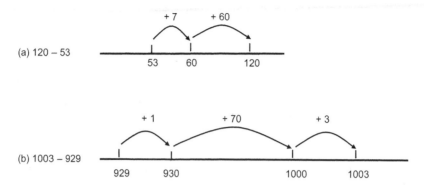

Figure 2.4   Finding (a) 120 - 53, (b) 1003 - 929

Strategy 5: For a subtraction, use an easier equivalent subtraction

If we think of subtraction as finding the difference between two numbers, then it should be obvious that you don't change the difference between two numbers if you add the same thing to both of them, or subtract the same thing from both of them. We can exploit this to simplify subtractions.

For the fluid balance calculation in Statement 10 in *Spot the errors* at the start of the chapter we had to find 2718 – 2035, which is the difference between 2718 and 2035. If we subtract 2000 from each of these numbers then we get an equivalent difference: 718 – 35. Instantly the calculation looks easier! We could then subtract 5 from both numbers and it becomes: 713 – 30, which is even easier.

Similarly, we can sometimes simplify subtractions by adding the same number to the two numbers, to get an equivalent difference. For example, to calculate 167 – 99, add 1 to both numbers and it becomes 168 – 100. Which is really easy!

Strategy 6: Use compensation

Compensation is a neat little trick that can be used for adding or subtracting numbers that are close to a multiple of 10, or 100. It works like this: to add, say, 49 to a number, add 50 (which is much easier to do) and then compensate for the fact that you have an added an extra 1 by subtracting it. For example, to find 137 + 49, do 137 + 50 = 187, then subtract 1 to get the answer, 186. All done mentally, of course!

Similarly, to find 2000 – 98, think 2000 – 100 = 1900. But we have subtracted 2 more than was required, so we *add* the 2 back on, to get the result 1902.

EXAMPLE 2.5

(a) A pharmacist has counted out 56 tablets of Drug A and adds a further 28 tablets. How many tablets are there now? We have to calculate 56 + 28.

Because 28 is close to 30, add 30 then compensate. Now, 56 + 30 = 86. But we have added an extra 2 here, so now take the 2 away, to give the result 84.

(b   An infusion is set to run for 480 minutes. After 97 minutes, how much longer has it to run? We have to calculate 480 – 97.

Because 97 is close to 100, subtract 100 and then compensate. Now, 480 – 100 = 380. But we have subtracted an extra 3 here, so we add it back on, to give the result, 383. The infusion has 383 minutes left to run. And you should have used less than one of these minutes to work this out!

We cannot resist showing you what compensation looks like when shown on an empty number-line diagram, because it makes it so easy to see what's going on. Figure 2.5 illustrates the calculations in Example 2.5. So, in (a) to add 28 we jump forward 30 and then step back 2. In (b) to subtract 97 we jump back 100 and then step forward 3.

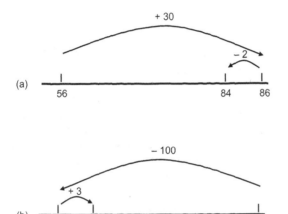

Figure 2.5   Using compensation in Example 2.5 to find (a) 56 + 28, (b) 480 – 97

Strategy 7: Start with friendlier numbers

The essence of this strategy is: if you don't like a particular calculation, do a different one that you do like! For example, if you were given 742 – 145, you might think to yourself, '742 – 142' would have been an easier question, because the numbers involved are so much friendlier! So, do that subtraction instead, and then adjust the answer as necessary: 742 – 142 = 600; and then we need to subtract a further 3 to get the result that 742 – 145 = 597. This is really just an extension of the compensation strategy.

EXAMPLE 2.6

(a) On a fluid balance chart the total output from midnight up to 5 am is 328 millilitres. In the next hour there is a further output of 175 millilitres of urine. So to calculate the total output up to 6 am we need to find 328 + 175.

(Continued)

(Continued)

A calculation with friendlier numbers would have been 325 + 175 = 500.

But for 328 rather than 325 we need an additional 3.

So, 328 + 175 = 503. So, the total output recorded at 6 am is 503 millilitres.

(b) To find the difference between a patient's total fluid intake of 1819 millilitres and their total fluid output of 1523 millilitres, we need to calculate 1819 – 1523.

A calculation with friendlier numbers would have been 1819 – 1519 = 300.

But for 1523 rather than 1519 we have to subtract a further 4.

So, 1819 – 1523 = 300 – 4 = 296.

How is addition done by a formal written method?

The principle of exchange

(a) As we move from right to left from units to tens to hundreds, and so on, ten in any place can be exchanged for one in the next.

(b) As we move from left to right, one in any place can be exchanged for ten in the next.

Given all these mental strategies, you should find that you rarely need to resort to a formal written method for addition. It might be necessary for numbers with four digits, for example – although you do always have the sensible option of using a calculator (see Chapter 7) – or for decimal numbers with different numbers of digits after the decimal point (see Chapter 9).

As an example, we will explain the method known as 'column addition' for 2097 + 586, as shown in Figure 2.6. A key principle of place value underlies this process: as we move from right to left, ten in one place are exchanged for one in the next place.

	(a)		(b)		(c)		(d)
	2 0 9 7		2 0 9 7		2 0 9 7		2 0 9 7
+	5 8 6	+	5 8 6	+	5 8 6	+	5 8 6
			3		8 3		2 6 8 3
			1		1 1		1 1

Figure 2.6 Column addition for 2097 + 586

Figure 2.6(a) shows how the addition is set up correctly. Note that the units-digits in the numbers (the 7 and the 6) are carefully placed in the same column; likewise the tens-digits (the 9 and the 8) and the hundreds-digits (the 0 and the 5). Only the top number has a thousands-digit (the 2). This lining up of the digits is absolutely crucial, because we need to ensure that we add units to units, tens to tens, and so on. In this column addition method we start by adding the units and work from right to left along the columns.

In Figure 2.6(b) we have added the 7 units and 6 units, giving 13 units. Ten of these can be exchanged for 1 in the tens-column. So we 'carry' this 1 into the next column, by writing it under the bottom line of the calculation. This leaves 3 in the units column, which is written in the answer space.

In (c) we have added the tens: 9 + 8 + the 1 that we carried = 18. Ten of these are exchanged for 1 in the next column, leaving 8 in the answer space.

In (d) we have added the hundreds: 0 + 5 + the 1 that we carried = 6. This is written in the answer space. And finally we have the 2 thousands in the top number to add to the answer space, giving the result of the addition: 2683.

This formal written method might be particularly useful when you have to find the total of more than two numbers.

EXAMPLE 2.7

A patient's fluid intake from midnight up to 6 pm is recorded on a fluid balance chart as 1897 ml. In the next hour the patients drinks 75 millilitres of water, receives 83 millilitres of fluid by infusion and receives 125 millilitres of fluid in intravenous medication. So to find the total fluid intake up to 7 pm the calculation required is 1897 + 75 + 83 + 125. Figure 2.7 shows how this might be done by column addition, to give the total to be recorded as 2180 millilitres.

$$
\begin{array}{r}
1\,8\,9\,7 \\
7\,5 \\
8\,3 \\
1\,2\,5 \\
\hline
2\,1\,8\,0 \\
\hline
1\,2\,2
\end{array}
$$

Figure 2.7   Column addition for 1897 + 75 + 83 + 125 (Example 2.7)

Notice again in Figure 2.7 how the digits are carefully arranged in columns, with the units lined up, the tens lined up, and so on. The sum of the units (7 + 5 + 3 + 5) is 20; so we carry 2 into the tens column, leaving 0 units recorded in the answer. Adding the tens (9 + 7 + 8 + 2 + 2) gives 28, which is 2 carried into the hundreds column and 8 recorded in the answer. Then adding the hundreds (8 + 1 + 2) gives 11, which is 1 carried into the thousands column and 1 recorded in the answer. Finally we add the thousands (1 plus the 1 below the line = 2), giving the total as 2180.

What about column subtraction?

If you know a formal written method for subtraction and you are confident with it, then you might sometimes want to use this for some of the trickier calculations you might encounter. We are not going to attempt to explain such a method here, because what we really think is that if you cannot do a subtraction easily by any of the informal strategies we have outlined above, then you might be well advised to turn to your calculator.

Even subtractions that look challenging can usually be done by bridging the gap. For example, to find 2125 – 578 use Strategy 4: adding on from 578, a step of 22 gets to 600, another 1500 gets to 2100, and a final step of 25 gets to 2125; which gives 22 + 1500 + 25 = 1547.

As we have pointed out earlier in this chapter, this applies especially to the subtractions with zeros in the first number, which are often the most difficult when you try to use a formal method. For example, to find 1003 – 488 use Strategy 5: add 12 to both numbers and you get the equivalent subtraction, 1015 – 500, which you can probably do in your head.

Use the questions in this check-up to practise the various strategies and methods outlined in this chapter. So, put the calculator away!

2.1   (a) What is the total cost of two items of IT equipment costing £800 and £700?

(b) What is the difference between £15 000 and £8000?

2.2   Practise some simple mental addition and subtraction:

(a) 65 + 7   (b) 18 + 17

(c) 82 + 18   (d) 107+ 49

(e) 83 + 75   (f) 50 – 13

(g) 92 – 9   (h) 57 – 49

(i) 103 – 7   (j) 105 – 97

2.3   Use the number-line diagrams in Figure 2.8 to calculate

(a) 127 + 39   (b) 217 – 148.

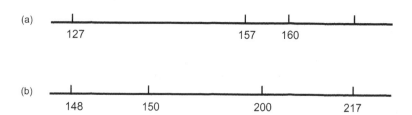

Figure 2.8   Empty number line diagrams for (a) 127 + 39, (b) 217 – 148 (check-up question 2.3)

2.4   Calculate mentally:

(a) 538 + 294 by partitioning the numbers into hundreds, tens and ones;

(b) 423 + 98 using compensation;

(c) 394 + 307 using 400 as a stepping-stone;

(d) 297 + 304 by any method that seems appropriate.

2.5   Calculate mentally:

(a) 1000 – 448, using compensation;

(b) 719 – 520 by making one of the numbers friendlier;

(c) 725 – 487, by adding on from 487, using 490, 500 and 700 as stepping-stones;

(d) 7020 – 6994 by adding 6 to both numbers;

(e) 5000 – 17, by any appropriate method.

2.6   You can check the answer to a subtraction by adding the answer to the second number in the subtraction, to see if you get back to the first number. For example, 28 – 15 = 13. Check: 13 + 15 = 28. Check all your answers to check-up question 2.5 in this way.

2.7   Find and correct any errors in the following calculations:

(a) 396 + 172 = 4168

(b) 405 – 144 = 361

(c) 1897 + 466 = 2363

(d) 3003 – 749 = 2366

2.8   Figure 2.9 shows the last few lines of a fluid balance chart for an adult patient. The running totals (in millilitres) for fluid intake and output up to 20:00 are given as 1963 and 1525. By 21:00 there have been additional intakes of 75 and 83, and an additional output of 120. Use this data to complete (a) the total intake up to 21:00, and (b) the total output up to 21:00.

Use the other information in the table to find the totals required in (c), (d), (e), (f), (g) and (h).

Find the difference between the final total for input and output (g) and (h). This is the fluid balance for the day. This is a positive balance if (g) is greater than (h) and a negative balance if (g) is less than (h).

Time	Intake (millilitres)				Output (millilitres)			
	Oral	IV	Other	Total	Urine	Oral	Other	Total
20:00		83		1963		150		1525
21:00	75	83		(a)			120	(b)
22:00		83	25	(c)	370			(d)
23:00		83		(e)				(f)
24:00		83		(g)			50	(h)

Figure 2.9   Part of a fluid balance chart (check-up question 2.8)

MULTIPLICATION AND DIVISION SKILLS

3

OBJECTIVES

The practitioner should be able to:

- recognize and use correctly four fundamental properties of multiplication and division
- recall instantly the product of two whole numbers from 1 to 10
- multiply or divide mentally a whole number or a decimal number by 10, 100 or 1000
- use knowledge of multiplications facts for multiplications and divisions involving multiples of 10, 100 or 1000
- use a range of mental and informal strategies for multiplication and division, appropriate to the numbers involved
- give the result of a division with a remainder when appropriate
- apply accurately an appropriate written method for doing a multiplication involving several digits
- use the method of short division for a whole number with any number of digits divided by a single-digit whole number

SPOT THE ERRORS

Identify any obvious errors in the following 12 statements. Do not use a calculator. You should not need to use a written method for the calculations involved in these statements.

1 The cost of 250 items at £67 each is the same as the cost of 67 items at £250 each.

2 There are 7 days in a week, 24 hours in a day and 60 minutes in an hour. So the number of minutes in a week is $(7 \times 24) \times 60$. This is also equal to $7 \times (24 \times 60)$.

3 To find 998×7, because 998 is 2 less than 1000, then 998×7 is $7000 - 2 = 6998$.

4 To divide a dose of 500 milligrams into 4 equal doses, the calculation required is $500 \div 4 = 125$. This result is correct because $125 \times 4 = 500$.

5 A prescription for 6 tablets a day for a week requires 42 tablets in total.

6 $7.05 \times 10 = 70.5$ and $70.5 \div 10 = 7.05$.

7 $83 \div 1000 = 0.830$.

8 7 hours is $7 \times 60 = 420$ minutes.

9 4 boxes of 28 tablets contain altogether $(4 \times 20) + (4 \times 8) = 80 + 32 = 112$ tablets.

10 $125 \times 24 = 125 \times 4 \times 6 = 500 \times 6 = 3000$.

11 $27 \div 5$ is equal to 5, remainder 2; so $27 \div 5 = 5.2$.

12 Factors of 8 are: 8, 16, 24, 32, 40, 48, and so on ...

(errors identified over the page)

ERRORS IDENTIFIED

The obvious errors are in Statements 3, 7, 11 and 12

Statement 3

To use the fact that 998 is just 2 less than 1000 in this multiplication, the 2 also has to be multiplied by 7, as follows: $998 \times 7 = (1000 - 2) \times 7 = (1000 \times 7) - (2 \times 7) = 7000 - 14 = 6986$. This is explained below using the fundamental property of multiplication and division that we call Property 3.

Statement 7

We explain later that to divide 83 by 1000 we have to move each digit in 83 three places to the right (or, to put it another way, shift the decimal point three places to the left). In the (incorrect) answer given in Statement 7 the digits (or the decimal point) have moved only two places. The correct result is $83 \div 1000 = 0.083$.

Statement 11

The first part is correct: $27 \div 5$ is equal to 5, remainder 2. But this does not mean the same thing as 5.2! To find $27 \div 5$ we could double both numbers to get $54 \div 10$, which is equal to 5.4. Strategies like this are outlined and explained in this chapter.

Statement 12

The numbers listed are the multiples of 8. The factors of 8 are numbers that divide exactly into 8: 1, 2, 4 and 8. In this chapter we explain how we can make use of factors when doing mental multiplications.

In this chapter we have a similar aim to that in Chapter 2: to encourage you to develop your mental and informal written methods of doing multiplication and division, making use of whatever number facts you know and with which you are confident. As in Chapter 2 most of what we do here is to make explicit the kinds of mental strategies that numerate people employ as a matter of course. We will also explain some written methods for multiplication and division, which you can resort to when necessary.

Note that this chapter is mainly about multiplication and division with whole numbers, although some of the objectives here do extend to decimal numbers. Further methods for multiplication and division involving decimal numbers are explained in Chapter 9. Some of the simple healthcare examples used in this chapter to illustrate multiplication and division techniques refer to units of measurement (like millilitres and milligrams) that are explained in later chapters, but we reckon you should be able to make sense of the examples without yet having studied these later chapters.

What are the fundamental properties of multiplication and division?

In order to explain a range of mental and written methods for doing multiplication and division calculations, we need to make explicit some fundamental mathematical laws that relate to these operations. We hope that you will recognize here ideas that you use already when you are doing calculations informally.

Property 1: You can swap the order of two numbers being multiplied together

This would mean, for example, that $12 \times 5 = 5 \times 12$. This is not immediately obvious. If you imagine 5 bags of 12 counters and 12 bags of 5 counters there does not seem any particular reason why they must contain the same number of counters. But the reason becomes clear when the multiplication is represented by a rectangular array, as shown in Figure 3.1. Here you can look at the 60 counters as either 5 (horizontal) rows of 12, or 12 (vertical) rows of 5. So clearly 12 fives is equal to 5 twelves.

Property 1:

If you know …

$7 \times 8 = 56$

then you also know:

$8 \times 7 = 56$

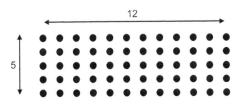

Figure 3.1   5 rows of 12 counters or 12 rows of 5 counters

This property is not just fundamental, but also useful. Many of us would find it easier to calculate 14 fives rather than 5 fourteens – because we find counting in fives easier than counting in fourteens. Also, it cuts down the number of separate results we have to learn in the multiplication tables; for example, if we know 9×8 then we also know 8×9. Look back at Statement 1 in *Spot the errors* at the start of this chapter; this is correct because it is using Property 1: $250 \times 67 = 67 \times 250$.

EXAMPLE 3.1

A common example of a rectangular array is the arrangement of tablets in some blister packs. A blister packet of 14 atenolol tablets has 2 rows of 7 tablets; or, to look at it another way, 7 rows of 2 tablets. This illustrates that 2 × 7 = 7 × 2.

Property 1 does *not* apply to division! For example, 5 ÷ 14 is not the same thing as 14 ÷ 5. It is crucial, therefore, when doing a division calculation on a calculator, to make sure you enter the numbers in the right order.

Property 2: When there are three numbers multiplied together it makes no difference which two you choose to multiply together first

Property 2: it's your choice ...

to find 5 × 8 × 7 you can choose either (5 × 8) × 7 or 5 × (8 × 7)

This would mean, for example, that 4 × 5 × 6 could mean either (4 × 5) × 6 or 4 × (5 × 6). where the brackets mean 'do this first'. Check this: (4 × 5) × 6 = 20 × 6 = 120; and 4 × (5 × 6) = 4 × 30 = 120. This property is really useful in mental strategies for multiplication, as we shall see below.

Look back at Statement 2 in *Spot the errors* at the start of this chapter; this is correct because it is using Property 2: (7 × 24) × 60 = 7 × (24 × 60).

Property 2 also does not apply to division. For example, (48 ÷ 8) ÷ 2 is *not* equal to 48 ÷ (8 ÷ 2). Check this for yourself. So we should never write a string of divisions, like 48 ÷ 8 ÷ 2, without brackets, because we could get two different results depending on which division we did first.

Property 3: You can 'distribute' a multiplication or a division across an addition or subtraction

To give a very simple example, this property would mean that (10 + 2) × 5 is equal to 10 × 5 added to 2 × 5. The multiplication by 5 has been distributed across the sum of 10 and 2. In Figure 3.2 we show how the array for 12 × 5 from Figure 3.1 can be seen as (10 + 2) × 5 and therefore split into two arrays of 10 × 5 and 2 × 5. This is a really important property that we require to do calculations involving multiplication or division, as we shall explain later in this chapter.

Multiplication distributed across subtraction would mean, for example, that (10 − 2) × 5 is equal to 10 × 5 subtract 2 × 5. The reader should check that these are correct:

(10 + 2) × 5 = (10 × 5) + (2 × 5)

(10 − 2) × 5 = (10 × 5) − (2 × 5)

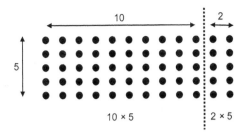

Figure 3.2 Showing that $(12 \times 5) = (10 \times 5) + (2 \times 5)$

Because of Property 2 we could also write these results with the multiplications reversed as follows:

$5 \times (10 + 2) = (5 \times 10) + (5 \times 2)$

$5 \times (10 - 2) = (5 \times 10) - (5 \times 2)$

The reader should check that these are correct. See also the error in Statement 3 in *Spot the errors*, and its correction. The examples in the box are the kinds of calculations we can do using Property 3 that we explain later in this chapter.

For division distributed across an addition, Property 3 would mean, for example, that $(30 + 6) \div 3$ would equal $30 \div 3$ added to $6 \div 3$. We have 'distributed' the 'divide by 3' across the addition of 30 and 6. For division distributed across a subtraction it would mean, for example, that $(30 - 6) \div 3$ would equal $30 \div 3$ subtract $6 \div 3$. Again, we suggest that you check these:

$(30 + 6) \div 3 = (30 \div 3) + (6 \div 3)$

$(30 - 6) \div 3 = (30 \div 3) - (6 \div 3)$

One last warning: you cannot reverse the divisions here, because Property 1 does not apply to division. So, for example, $3 \div (30 + 6)$ is *not* equal to $(3 \div 30) + (3 \div 6)$.

> **Property 3: examples**
>
> Multiplication distributed over ...
>
> addition
> $98 \times 3 = (90 + 8) \times 3$
> $= (90 \times 3) + (8 \times 3)$
> $= 270 + 24 = 294$
>
> subtraction
> $98 \times 3 = (100 - 2) \times 3$
> $= (100 \times 3) - (2 \times 3)$
> $= 300 - 6 = 294$

Property 4: Division is the inverse of multiplication

In mathematics two operations are called inverses if one undoes the effect of the other. Figure 3.3, for example, shows, by starting the loop at the 15, how the effect of multiplying by 6 is undone by dividing by 6; and, by starting at the 90, how the effect of dividing by 6 is undone by multiplying by 6. This means that when we are faced with a division, say $a \div b$, then the question we ask ourselves is: 'By what do we multiply b to get a? So, given $120 \div 10$ we could ask: 'By what do we multiply 10 to get 120? Answer: 12.

Apart from anything else this is a useful way of checking that the result of a division calculation is correct. For example, if we calculate $675 \div 9$ and get the result 75, then we can check whether or not this is correct by multiplying 75 by 9 and

> **Property 4:**
>
> **if you know . . .**
> $7 \times 8 = 56$
> then you also know:
> $56 \div 8 = 7$
> $56 \div 7 = 8$

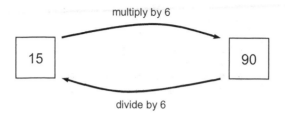

Figure 3.3 Multiplying by 6 and dividing by 6 are inverse operations

seeing if we get back to 675. This is an important process in practice for checking dosage calculations. See also the use of multiplication to check a division in the correct Statement 4 in *Spot the errors*.

What are the prerequisites for being able to do multiplication and division calculations?

There are two important prerequisites for being able to deal confidently and efficiently with multiplication and division calculations.

Product

The result of multiplying together two numbers is called their *product*. For example, the product of 7 and 8 is 56.

Prerequisite 1: You must be able to recall instantly the product of any two whole numbers from 1 to 10

In other words, you should know by heart all the multiplication tables up to 10 × 10, as shown in Figure 3.4. To show how to read the results in this grid we have highlighted 7 × 8 and 8 × 7.

×	1	2	3	4	5	6	7	8	9	10
1	1	2	3	4	5	6	7	8	9	10
2	2	4	6	8	10	12	14	16	18	20
3	3	6	9	12	15	18	21	24	27	30
4	4	8	12	16	20	24	28	32	36	40
5	5	10	15	20	25	30	35	40	45	50
6	6	12	18	24	30	36	42	48	54	60
7	7	14	21	28	35	42	49	56	63	70
8	8	16	24	32	40	48	56	64	72	80
9	9	18	27	36	45	54	63	72	81	90
10	10	20	30	40	50	60	70	80	90	100

Figure 3.4 Multiplication tables up to 10 × 10 (7 × 8 and 8 × 7 highlighted)

To help you to reinforce your knowledge of these, we have a few suggestions. First, copy the headings for rows and columns in the grid shown in Figure 3.4 and then fill in all the results for yourself, working from left to right, row by row. Then jumble up the order of the headings for the rows and columns and fill in all the results again. See, for example, Figure 3.5, where we have put in a few products, leaving the rest for the reader to complete. Do this over and over again until you can just write in all the results without hesitation.

×	2	7	6	9	1	5	4	3	8	10
7								21		
5										
3										
1	2	7	6							
2										
4										
9						45				
8										
10										100
6										

Figure 3.5   To reinforce knowledge of multiplication facts complete tables like this

Our second suggestion is to exploit all the patterns and relationships in the multiplication tables. Most people know their 5-times and 10-times tables because the patterns are so clear, as can be seen in the columns headed 5 and 10 in Figure 3.4. But look also at the column for the 9-times table. Notice that as the unit digit decreases by 1 each time the tens digit increases by 1. So the two digits in the numbers in the 9-times table from 9 to 90 always add up to 9.

Here's a little trick for the 9-times table. Put your ten fingers flat on the table and mentally number them 1 to 10 from left to right. If you want 7×9, bend back finger number 7; you can now see 6 fingers to the left of the bent finger and 3 to the right. That tells you that the result is 63. This works for multiplying 9 by any number from 1 to 10.

Get into the habit of using what you know confidently to work out what you are unsure of. For example, if you cannot remember 6×8, then think of it as 5 eights plus another eight, so that's $40 + 8 = 48$. This is an example of using Property 3 above, distributing the multiplication by 8 across the addition of 5 and 1:

$$6 \times 8 = (5 + 1) \times 8 = (5 \times 8) + (1 \times 8) = 40 + 8 = 48.$$

If you are unsure about 7×6, recall that 7×3 is 21 and double it to get $7 \times 6 = 42$.

Knowing the 7-times table is particularly important because there are 7 days in a week.

EXAMPLE 3.2

How many tablets are required for a week's prescription of (a) 2 tablets a day, (b) 3 tablets a day, (c) 4 tablets a day, and so on.

(a) $2 \times 7 = 14$ tablets; (b) $3 \times 7 = 21$ tablets; (c) $4 \times 7 = 28$ tablets

and so on: $5 \times 7 = 35$ tablets, $6 \times 7 = 42$ tablets ...

Good knowledge of the multiplication tables enables you to use the idea that division is the inverse of multiplication (Property 4 above) in many practical situations.

EXAMPLE 3.3

(a) A patient requires 40 milligrams of prednisolone as a daily dose. Prednisolone is available in 5-milligram tablets as stock. How many tablets should be given? (Milligrams are explained in Chapter 6.)

The calculation required is $40 \div 5$, meaning 'how many 5s make 40?' In the 5-times table we recall $5 \times 8 = 40$, so 8 tablets should be given.

(b) A dose of erythromycin is to be given to a patient four times a day. What is the time interval between each dose?

There are 24 hours in a day, so the calculation required is $24 \div 4$, which can be thought of as 'what multiplied by 4 gives 24?' In the 4-times table we recall $4 \times 6 = 24$, so $24 \div 4 = 6$. The drug should be administered at 6-hourly intervals.

Prerequisite 2: You must know how to multiply or divide mentally a whole number (or a decimal number) by 10, 100 or 1000

Because of the base-ten, place-value principles that underpin our number system (see Chapter 1), multiplication and division by 10 and powers of 10 are really very simple, but also fundamental to both mental and written calculations.

First, we note what happens when we multiply a number of units by 10. For example, $7 \times 10 = 70$. All that has happened is that the 7 units have become 7 tens.

If we now multiply this by 10, we get $70 \times 10 = 700$; the 7 tens have now become 7 hundreds. And so on. So, when we multiply a number by 10, the units become tens, the tens become hundreds, the hundreds become thousands, and so on. So all the digits move one place to the left, as illustrated in Figure 3.6(a), where 4567 is multiplied by 10: the 4 thousands become 4 ten-thousands; the 5 hundreds become 5 thousands; the 6 tens become 6 hundreds; and the 7 units become 7 tens. The final zero in the result, 45 670, is required as a place-holder.

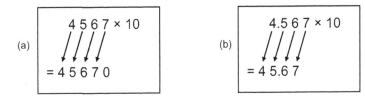

Figure 3.6   When multiplying by 10 each digit moves one place to the left

Because the principle of place value works exactly the same way to the right of the decimal point, multiplication by 10 works just the same with decimal numbers, as shown in Figure 3.6(b), where 4.567 is multiplied by 10: the 4 ones become 4 tens; the 5 tenths become 5 units; the 6 hundredths become 6 tenths; and the 7 thousandths become 7 hundredths. So, 4.567 × 10 = 45.67.

Another way of describing what happens when you multiply by 10 is to say that the *decimal point* moves one place to the right. Often it is easier to visualize the decimal point moving rather than the digits, as shown in the following examples.

Multiplication and division by 10

× 10: move each digit one place to the left; or move the decimal point one place to the right.
÷ 10: move each digit one place to the right; or move the decimal point one place to the left.

EXAMPLE 3.4

(a) One bottle of albumin solution provides 4.5 milligrams of albumin. To find how much will be provided in 10 bottles we have to calculate 4.5 × 10. Moving the decimal point one place to the right gives 4.5 × 10 = 45; so the result is 45 milligrams.

(b) One tablet contains 0.025 grams of atenolol. So, 10 tablets will contain 0.025 × 10 grams, which, by moving the decimal point one place to the right, equals 0.25 grams.

Because division is the inverse of multiplication, dividing by 10 has the reverse effect: each digit is moved one place to the right, as illustrated in Figure 3.7. In (a) 6789 is divided by 10 to give 678.9; in (b) 6.789 is divided by 10 to give 0.6789. Note in (b) that we place a zero before the decimal point when there are no units (see Chapter 1). Again it is often easier to think of the decimal point moving, in this case one place to the left.

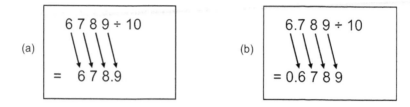

Figure 3.7 When dividing by 10 each digit moves one place to the right

---

EXAMPLE 3.5

(a) A dose of 10 millilitres of Calpol® contains 240 milligrams of paracetamol. So the number of milligrams of paracetamol in 1 millilitre is 240 ÷ 10. To divide by 10 each digit in 240 moves one place to the right, giving 24.0; we can drop the trailing zero after the decimal point, giving the result 24 milligrams. (We explain concentrations like this in more detail in Chapter 12.)

(b) An oral suspension contains 0.25 grams of ampicillin in 10 millilitres. So the dosage in 1 millilitre will be 0.25 ÷ 10 (grams). To divide 0.25 by 10 we move the decimal point one place to the left, giving 0.025 (grams).

Multiplication and division by 100

× 100: move the digits two places to the left; or move the decimal point two places to the right.
÷ 100: move the digits two places to the right; or move the decimal point two places to the left.

Multiplying a number by 100 is equivalent to multiplying by 10 and then multiplying by 10 again. So each digit moves two places to the left (so the decimal point moves two places to the right). It follows that when we divide by 100 each digit moves two places to the right (so the decimal point moves two places to the left). Similarly multiplying or dividing by 1000 will involve digits (or the decimal point) moving three places. Here are some examples to show how all this works:

7.5 × 100 = 750	7.5 × 1000 = 7500	7.5 ÷ 100 = 0.075
0.025 × 100 = 2.5	0.025 × 1000 = 25	250 ÷ 1000 = 0.25
2 ÷ 100 = 0.02	2 ÷ 1000 = 0.002	0.2 × 1000 = 200
1050 ÷ 1000 = 1.05	105 ÷ 100 = 1.05	0.105 × 100 = 10.5

Multiplying and dividing by 10, 100 and, especially, 1000, are important processes in converting measurements between units (such as millilitres to litres, or grams to milligrams), as we shall see in Chapters 4–6.

How do you use knowledge of multiplications facts to multiply by multiples of 10, 100 or 1000?

We now want to make sure that you can do mentally simple multiplications involving multiples of 10, 100 or 1000, such as 8×60, 4×200, 5×4000.

EXAMPLE 3.6

An infusion is set to run for 8 hours. How many minutes is that? There are 60 minutes in an hour, so the number of minutes is 8×60. Because $60 = 6 \times 10$ the calculation required is $8 \times (6 \times 10)$, which, using what we have called above Property 2, is equal to $(8 \times 6) \times 10 = 48 \times 10 = 480$.

In the example above we have given a long-winded explanation of why you can do this: to multiply by 60, multiply by 6 and then multiply by 10. In the same way, to multiply by 600 we could multiply by 6 and then multiply by 100. And, likewise, '$\times$ 6000' can be done in two steps, '$\times$ 6' and then '$\times$ 1000'. So, if we know $8 \times 6 = 48$, we also know $8 \times 60 = 480$, $8 \times 600 = 4800$, and $8 \times 6000 = 48\ 000$.

If you know ...

$7 \times 8 = 56$

then you also know:

$70 \times 8 = 560$

$7 \times 80 = 560$

$700 \times 8 = 5600$

$70 \times 800 = 56\ 000$

and so on.

It should then be pretty obvious what to do with 80×60. This is $(8 \times 10) \times 60$, which is equal to $8 \times (10 \times 60)$, so equal to 8×600, which we know is 4800. If you are thinking that all you have to do is collect up the zeros from these multiples of 10 and stick them on the end of the answer, you are right. So, for 800×60, we do $8 \times 6 = 48$ and then stick on the three zeros we took from the 800 and the 60, to get the result $48\ 000$.

But just be a little careful when the multiplication produces one or more additional zeros …

EXAMPLE 3.7

A patient is given 500 milligrams of erythromycin orally 4 times a day for 5 days. That amounts to 20 doses over this period. The total number of milligrams of the drug received in this time is 500×20. To calculate this, we can drop the three zeros and find $5 \times 2 = 10$; then putting back the three zeros we get the result to be $10\ 000$ milligrams. (We explain in Chapter 6 that this would normally be written as 10 grams.) There are four zeros altogether in this result, but one of these came from 5×2.

How do you mentally multiply a 2-digit number by a single-digit number?

A numerate person should be able to calculate mentally – perhaps supported by a few jottings – the product of a two-digit number and a single-digit number, such as 28×6 or 72×8. Often they will be able to do this for a three-digit number as well. The most obvious strategy is to partition the two-digit number into tens and units (or in the case of a three-digit number, hundreds, tens and units), and then to use Property 3 to distribute the multiplication across the addition.

EXAMPLE 3.8

(a) Many tablets come in packets of 28, so pharmacists often find themselves multiplying 28 by 2, 3, 4, 5, 6, and so on. How many tablets are there in 6 packets of 28? We need 28×6. The number 28 is $20 + 8$. So, using Property 3, to multiply 28 by 6 you can multiply the 20 by 6 and multiply the 8 by 6, and then add the results:

$28 \times 6 = (20 + 8) \times 6 = (20 \times 6) + (8 \times 6) = 120 + 48 = 168.$

(b) An infusion is set to deliver 83 millilitres each hour. So the number of millilitres that have been delivered after 6 hours is 83×6. To calculate this mentally think of it as 80×6 add 3×6, which is $480 + 18 = 498$ (millilitres).

The calculation in Example 3.8(a) can also be done using subtraction. We could think of the 28 as $30 - 2$. Then to multiply 28 by 6 we can multiply 30 by 6 and 2 by 6 and then subtract the second answer from the first: $28 \times 6 = (30 - 2) \times 6 = (30 \times 6) - (2 \times 6) = 180 - 12 = 168$. Using subtraction is a good option when the two-digit (or three-digit number) is just less than a multiple of 10, as in this case where 28 is only 2 short of 30.

Below are some more examples of these techniques. We have written out the reasoning in full, but most of this will be done mentally:

$23 \times 5 = (20 + 3) \times 5 = (20 \times 5) + (3 \times 5) = 100 + 15 = 115$

$72 \times 8 = (70 + 2) \times 8 = (70 \times 8) + (2 \times 8) = 560 + 16 = 576$

$125 \times 3 = (100 + 20 + 5) \times 3 = (100 \times 3) + (20 \times 3) + (5 \times 3) = 300 + 60 + 15 = 375$

$49 \times 4 = (50 - 1) \times 4 = (50 \times 4) - (1 \times 4) = 200 - 4 = 196$

$198 \times 3 = (200 - 2) \times 3 = (200 \times 3) - (2 \times 3) = 600 - 6 = 594.$

What are factors and how can they be used in mental multiplication?

Why did we finish up with 24 hours in a day? What's special about 24? Well, it is probably because 24 is a number that has several factors: these are numbers that divide exactly into 24. The number 24 can be written as the product of two numbers in these four ways: 1×24, 2×12, 3×8, 4×6. The numbers in these products are the factors of 24: 1, 2, 3, 4, 6, 8, 12 and 24. Because it has these factors we can easily split a period of 24 hours into: 2 periods of 12 hours; or 3 periods of 8 hours; or 4 periods of 6 hours; or 6 periods of 4 hours; or 8 periods of 3 hours; or 12 periods of 2 hours; or 24 periods of 1 hour.

An example: factors of 60

A factor of 60 is a number that divides exactly into 60. Factors of 60 are 1, 2, 3, 4, 5, 6, 10, 12, 15, 20, 30, and 60.

There are particular numbers like 24 that we encounter frequently in practice, for which it is really useful to know their factors. In the box, for example, we have listed the factors of 60; these, like the factors of 24, are useful for calculations involving time.

It is really useful to know the different ways in which 10, 100 and 1000 can be written as the product of two factors:

10 is equal to 1×10, or 2×5;

100 is equal to 1×100, or 2×50, or 4×25, or 5×20, or 10×10;

1000 is equal to 1×1000, or 2×500, or 4×250, or 8×125, or 10×100, or 20×50, or 25×40.

Similarly, because numbers like 75, 250, 500, 750 turn up frequently in drug calculations, get used to thinking of them in terms of various factors, such as:

$75 = 3 \times 25$	$250 = 5 \times 50$	$250 = 2 \times 125$	$500 = 2 \times 250$
$500 = 4 \times 125$	$500 = 20 \times 25$	$750 = 3 \times 250$	$750 = 5 \times 150$.

Knowing these factors enables us to do some nifty mental calculations. For a start, whenever there is a 5 involved in a multiplication we will try to double it to make 10. Whenever we see a 25, for example, we will try to multiply it by 4, because this gives us 100. Here are three examples of what we mean:

(a) Calculate 360×5: think of the 360 as 180×2; this enables us to multiply the 5 by 2 which is bound to make the calculation easier. So $360 \times 5 = 180 \times 2 \times 5 = 180 \times 10 = 1800$.

(b) Calculate 24×25: think of the 24 as 6×4; this enables us to multiply the 25 by 4 which we enjoy doing! So $24 \times 25 = 6 \times 4 \times 25 = 6 \times 100 = 600$.

(c) Calculate 75×12: think of the 75 as 3×25 and the 12 as 4×3. Then $75 \times 12 = 3 \times 25 \times 4 \times 3 = 3 \times 100 \times 3 = 300 \times 3 = 900$.

EXAMPLE 3.9

(a) An infusion is delivering 25 units of heparin each minute. How many units are delivered in an hour? The calculation required is 25×60.

We would like to multiply the 25 by 4, so think of the 60 as 4×15.

The calculation is now $25 \times 4 \times 15 = 100 \times 15 = 1500$ units.

(b) An infusion is set to deliver 125 millilitres of a preparation each hour. How many millilitres are delivered in 24 hours? The calculation required is 125×24.

The 24 can helpfully be written as 4×6. The calculation then becomes $125 \times 4 \times 6 = 500 \times 6 = 3000$ millilitres.

There are many other ways in which we can exploit various relationships between numbers to deal with the calculations that arise in practice. We cannot cover all these here, but there will be more ideas to encourage you in mental calculation in the examples we use in subsequent chapters.

Are there any mental strategies for division calculations?

The first strategy for division is always to think of it as the inverse of multiplication. So, for example, given $3000 \div 6$, we think: 'What do we multiply by 6 to get 3000?' Well, we know $6 \times 5 = 30$, and therefore $6 \times 500 = 3000$, so $3000 \div 6 = 500$.

Equivalent divisions

You can change a division calculation to an equivalent calculation by multiplying or dividing both numbers by the same thing.

The second strategy is to use Property 3 to distribute the division across numbers you can deal with easily. For example, $176 \div 8$ could be thought of as $(160 + 16) \div 8$, which equals $(160 \div 8) + (16 \div 8) = 20 + 2 = 22$.

One more suggestion is to use the principle given in the accompanying box to simplify a division. Here are four examples:

(a) Calculate $34 \div 5$: multiply both numbers by 2 to get $68 \div 10 = 6.8$.

(b) Calculate $600 \div 300$: divide both numbers by 100 to get $6 \div 3 = 2$.

(c) Calculate $400 \div 16$: divide both numbers by 4 to get $100 \div 4 = 25$.

(d) Calculate $600 \div 25$: multiply both numbers by 4 to get $2400 \div 100 = 24$.

EXAMPLE 3.10

An infusion is delivering 1500 units of heparin each hour. How many units are delivered in a minute? The calculation required is 1500 ÷ 60. Dividing both numbers by 10 this becomes 150 ÷ 6. Dividing both numbers by 3 this becomes 50 ÷ 2, which equals 25. So 25 units are delivered in a minute.

This idea of equivalent divisions is something we return to in Chapter 9 when we consider calculations with decimals. In particular, we shall see how to change a division involving decimal numbers into one that has only whole numbers. For example, multiplying both numbers in 0.2 ÷ 0.05 by 100 changes it 20 ÷ 5, which is easy. We also use this idea in discussing equivalent fractions and equivalent ratios in Chapter 11.

What about remainders?

When a division does not work out exactly, we sometimes (but not often) give the result with a *remainder*. For example, consider 20 ÷ 6; 20 is more than 3 × 6 (18), but less than 4 × 6 (24). So 20 is 3 × 6 plus an extra 2. We say that 20 ÷ 6 is equal to '3, remainder 2'.

EXAMPLE 3.11

A patient is prescribed 3 tablets of diazepam each day for 30 days. The total number of tablets required is therefore 90. Diazepam is supplied in packets of 28 tablets How many packets and how many additional tablets are required? The calculation is 90 ÷ 28.

Now 28 × 3 = 84, which is 6 short of 90. So 90 ÷ 28 = 3, remainder 6. This means that 3 packets and 6 additional tablets are required.

Most divisions in healthcare practice arise in the context of some kind of measurement. In these cases, it will not usually be appropriate to give a result with a remainder. Normally the division would continue beyond the decimal point, generating digits to whatever level of accuracy is required. The method of 'short division' to do this is explained later in this chapter.

What written method might be used for multiplication involving larger numbers?

Extending the idea of a rectangular array used in Figure 3.1, multiplication can be pictured as the area of a rectangle, as shown in Figure 3.8(a). The area of a rectangle is the amount of space inside, measured in square units. In this case the multiplication 5×12 is represented by a rectangle 5 units by 12 units, with an area of 60 square units. Extending this idea, any multiplication can be represented by the area of a rectangle, without drawing all the individual square units, as shown in Figure 3.8(b).

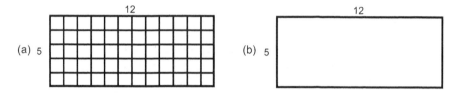

Figure 3.8   The area of these rectangles is $5 \times 12 = 60$ square units

So, as an example, consider 28×43. This can be represented by a rectangle, 28 units by 43, as shown in Figure 3.9(a) (not drawn to scale). In Figure 3.9(b) we have divided this into four sections by partitioning the 28 into $20 + 8$ and the 43 into $40 + 3$ (again not drawn to scale). This gives us four areas to calculate, all of which are simple mental calculations: 20×40 ($= 800$), 8×40 ($= 320$), 20×3 ($= 60$), and 8×3 (24). On the right of Figure 3.9 we have totalled these to get $28 \times 43 = 1204$.

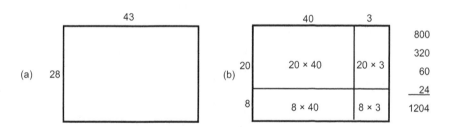

Figure 3.9   Calculating 28×43 using four areas

This is sometimes called the 'grid method'; we think it is a method for multiplication that is easy to carry out and to understand. Of course, if the reader is confident in using some other method, such as 'long multiplication', then that's fine!

Figure 3.10(a) and (b) are a couple more examples, including one with a three-digit number.

In (a) we find that 75×32 is equal to the sum of four areas: 70×30 ($= 2100$), 5×30 ($= 150$), 70×2 ($= 140$) and 5×2 ($=10$), giving $75 \times 32 = 2100 + 150 + 140 + 10 = 2400$.

In (b) we find that 243×25 is equal to the sum of six areas: 20×200 ($= 4000$), 5×200 ($= 1000$), 20×40 ($= 800$), 5×40 ($= 200$), 20×3 ($= 60$) and 5×3 ($= 15$), giving $243 \times 25 = 4000 + 1000 + 800 + 200 + 60 + 15 = 6075$.

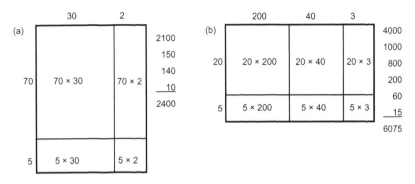

Figure 3.10   Using the grid method for (a) 75 × 32, (b) 243 × 25

With a bit of practice of this method, you will find that you can condense the written record considerably. For any multiplications more difficult than those in Figure 3.10, or if you are not confident with written methods at this level, then use a calculator!

How does short division work?

We reckon you should be able at least to divide a number with several digits by a single-digit number, using the method known as *short division*. Figure 3.11 shows the division of 252 by 7.

(a) 7 | 2 5 2   (b) 7 | 2²5 2

                 3   3 6
(c) 7 | 2²5⁴2   (d) 7 | 2²5⁴2

Figure 3.11   Dividing 252 by 7 using short division

We will explain the calculation in Figure 3.11 step by step.

Step (a): the calculation is set up to divide the 252 by the 7. The answer will appear above the horizontal line.

Step (b): the 2 (hundreds) cannot be divided by 7 without breaking the 2 hundreds down into 20 tens; this is done by writing a little 2 next to the 5 tens, indicating that we now have 25 tens.

Step (c): 25 divided by 7 is 3, remainder 4; the 3 is put in the tens position in the answer above the line; the remainder, 4, is carried to the units where it becomes 40 units, so we now have 42 in the units position.

Step (d): 42 divided by 7 is 6 exactly; the 6 is put in the answer above the line. The calculation is complete: 252 ÷ 7 = 36.

Figure 3.12 shows three further examples of short division.

$$
\text{(a)} \quad 3\,\overline{)\,7^1 5\,9}\;=\;253 \qquad \text{(b)} \quad 8\,\overline{)\,3^3 0^6 1^5 6}\;=\;377 \qquad \text{(c)} \quad 4\,\overline{)\,3^3 7\,5\!.^3 0^2 0}\;=\;93.75
$$

Figure 3.12   (a) 759 ÷ 3 = 253, (b) 3016 ÷ 8 = 377, (c) 375 ÷ 4 = 93.75

In (a) the steps involved are: 7 divided by 3 is 2 remainder 1; 15 divided by 3 is 5; 9 divided by 3 is 3.

In (b) the steps involved are: 30 divided by 8 is 3 remainder 6; 61 divided by 8 is 7 remainder 5; 56 divided by 8 is 7.

In (c) the division does not work out exactly as a whole number answer, and so it is continued by filling in extra zeros as necessary after the decimal point; the process is exactly the same beyond the decimal point. Further examples of division involving decimal numbers are given in Chapter 9.

We do not intend to attempt to explain the method known as 'long division'. Divisions more difficult than those we have given here would be probably best done on a calculator. See Chapter 7 on the use of calculators.

HAVE A CHECK-UP

Use the questions in this check-up to practise the various strategies and methods outlined in this chapter. No calculator needed!

3.1   Figure 3.13 shows just a small section cut out of a grid showing the products of the numbers 1 to 10, in order. Work out the missing numbers.

36		48	54
42	49		
48			72
54	63	72	81

Figure 3.13   What are the missing numbers in this section of a table of multiplication results? (check-up question 3.1)

3.2   (a) Write out the 7-times table from 7×1 to 7×10.
      (b) Which of these results would you use to find the total number of tablets
         required for a course of 1 tablet every 8 hours for a week?

3.3   Calculate: (a) 12×5

      (b) 50×8 (c) 25×12

      (d) 15×30 (e) 99×7

3.4   Calculate: (a) $600 \div 5$

      (b) $250 \div 25$ (c) $120 \div 24$

      (d) $96 \div 3$ (e) $360 \div 90$

3.5   A capsule contains 25 milligrams of Drug A. How many capsules would be
      required for a dosage of:

      (a) 100 milligrams?   (b) 175 milligrams?

3.6   Given that $73 \times 69 = 5037$, write down two divisions results involving the same
      numbers.

3.7   (a) Write out the 28-times table from 28×1 to 28×10.
      (b) Which of these results would you use to find how many packs of 28 tablets
         would be needed to supply 140 tablets?

3.8   (a) Complete the following: $100 \div 28 =$ ☐ remainder ☐.
      (b) How many packs of 28 and how many additional tablets would be required
         to supply 100 tablets?

3.9   A patient is prescribed 2 tablets of erythromycin orally every 6 hours for 14 days.

      (a) What is the total number of tablets required for the patient to complete the
         course of erythromycin?
      (b) How many packs of 28 tablets are required for this course of treatment?

3.10   An infusion delivers 83 millilitres per hour. How many millilitres would be
      delivered in 12 hours? (Calculation required: 83×12)

3.11   The strength of a solution of sodium chloride is 0.009 grams in 1 millilitre.
      How many grams would there be in 100 millilitres? (Calculation required:
      0.009×100)

3.12   A volume of 100 millilitres of a solution contains 1.8 grams of sodium chloride.
      How much would there be in 1 millilitre? (Calculation required: $1.8 \div 100$)

3.13   Use the grid method of multiplication (or some other non-calculator method)
      to find how much fluid is infused in 24 hours if 75 millilitres are infused each
      hour. (Calculation required: 75×24)

(Continued)

(Continued)

3.14   Do a multiplication to check whether this division is correct: $450 \div 25 = 16$.

3.15   Check the short divisions in Figure 3.14 and identify any errors.

$$\text{(a)}\ 6\ \overline{)\ 1^14^24\ 6}\quad\quad \frac{2\ 4\ 1}{}$$

(a) $6\overline{)1^14^24\ 6}$ with quotient $2\ 4\ 1$

(b) $5\overline{)1^11^22^25}$ with quotient $1\ 4\ 5$

(c) $4\overline{)9^17^10^20}$ with quotient $2\ 4\ 2.5$

(d) $8\overline{)6^65^10^20^40}$ with quotient $8.1\ 2\ 5$

Figure 3.14   Find any errors in these short divisions (check-up question 3.15)

UNITS OF LENGTH

4

OBJECTIVES

In a practical healthcare context the practitioner should be able to:

- make reasonable estimates of lengths in metres, centimetres and millimetres and have a sense of the magnitude of each of these units
- recall and use the relationships between metres, centimetres and millimetres
- use correctly the abbreviations for these units of length
- accurately read measurements of length using a variety of scales

SPOT THE ERRORS

Identify any obvious errors in the measurements of length used in the following eight statements.

1   The British Heart Foundation guidance is that the health of men is at risk if they have waist measurements over 94 cm and at high risk if they have waist measurements over 102 cm.

2   The body lengths of most newborn babies at full term in the UK lie within the range 450 to 560 millimetres.

3   The heights of most 2-year-old children in the UK lie in the range 79 to 95 centimetres.

4   A man who is 2 metres in height would be generally regarded as very tall.

5   There are 1000 metres in a millimetre.

6   1 centimetre is 0.01 of a metre.

7   25 millimetres is 2.5 centimetres and 0.025 metres.

8   Using the measuring scale in Figure 4.1 the length of the arrow is about 8.52 centimetres.

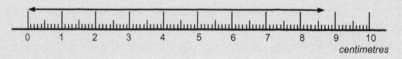

Figure 4.1   What is the approximate length of the arrow?

Are the errors you have spotted potentially serious in medical health practice?

(errors identified on page 52)

What units of length might be met in healthcare contexts?

This is the first of three chapters about units of measurement, covering length, liquid volume (Chapter 5) and weight (Chapter 6). Of these aspects of measurement, length is probably the least difficult to deal with and the one with the fewest applications in the context of healthcare practice. But we include it here because it is useful for underlining some key principles that will help in understanding the units that follow in subsequent chapters.

In the metric system units of length are all based on the *metre*. If an average man simultaneously looks in one direction and stretches out his arm to point in the opposite direction, the distance from his nose to his finger-tip is about a metre.

Other units of length are then obtained by adding *prefixes* to the word 'metre'. There are loads of these *prefixes* available. For example, the reader may have come across *mega* (a million) and *giga* (a thousand million) as prefixes for the amount of memory (measured in *megabytes* or *gigabytes*) on a computer; or you may hear people using the prefix *nano*, as in the very, very small time interval, the *nanosecond*. But you will be relieved to know that in healthcare practice normally only a few of these prefixes will be needed.

Two prefixes are commonly used to produce lengths smaller than a metre: *centi* (a hundredth of) to give the familiar and convenient *centimetre*, a hundredth of a metre, which is about the width of your little finger; and *milli*, to give the *millimetre*, a thousandth of a metre, which is about the thickness of a line drawn with a soft pencil. We will also use the less familiar and neglected *decimetre* (a tenth of a metre) – which is about the width of your hand – to enable us to explain how these prefixes work.

Some metric prefixes for making smaller units

deci means 'a tenth of'
centi means 'a hundredth of'
milli means 'a thousandth of'

So, metres, decimetres, centimetres and millimetres are some of the metric units used for measuring length. Working from left to right, each unit is equivalent to ten of the next one. A metre is 10 decimetres, a decimetre is 10 centimetres, and a centimetre is 10 millimetres.

This means, therefore, that, working from right to left, each unit is one tenth (0.1) of the previous one. A millimetre is 0.1 of a centimetre, a centimetre is 0.1 of a decimetre, a decimetre is 0.1 of a metre.

One other familiar prefix in the context of length is the prefix *kilo*, which means 'a thousand'. So, for example, a kilometre is 1000 metres. This prefix will feature strongly in Chapter 6, as the *kilogram* is an important unit of weight.

What are the standard abbreviations for these units of length?

There are accepted international conventions for all units of measurement. These are based on the *Systeme Internationale* (SI) and healthcare practitioners will encounter these frequently in charts, measuring scales, and labels on packets and bottles.

ERRORS IDENTIFIED

The obvious errors are Statements 5 and 8.

Statement 5

As we explain later in this chapter, the prefix 'milli' means 'one thousandth', so 1 millimetre is one thousandth of a metre. The statement is the wrong way round: there are 1000 millimetres in a metre. A thousand metres is actually a kilometre.

Statement 8

The length of the arrow in Figure 4.1 is about 8.7 centimetres. It clearly lies between 8 and 9 centimetres. The space between 8 and 9 is divided into 10 equal intervals by marks representing 8.1, 8.2, 8.3, 8.4, 8.5, 8.6, 8.7, 8.8 and 8.9. Each of these intervals is a tenth of a centimetre (0.1 cm). The mark drawn halfway between 8 and 9 represents 8.5 centimetres. The arrow looks longer than this by about 2 tenths of a centimetre, getting to about 8.7 on the scale. The 8.52 centimetres in Statement 8 is only 2 hundredths of a centimetre beyond 8.5, which is such a small distance beyond 8.5 that we probably would not notice it.

These errors are not likely to have serious consequences in a healthcare context, other than the embarrassment caused to the practitioner.

(now continue reading from page 51)

The abbreviation for *metre* is m (just one lower case letter). From this the other units of weight are constructed using prefixes, as mentioned above. The symbol for *deci* (a tenth) is d; that for *centi* (a hundredth) is c, and that for *milli* (a thousandth) is m; giving m, dm, cm and mm as the symbols for metre, decimetre, centimetre and millimetre respectively.

Note that the abbreviations for these three prefixes are lower case letters (d, c and m).

In healthcare practice these abbreviations will be used in relation to length mainly for body measurements such as height and waist measurements, and also encountered in the sizes of some medical resources, such as surgical dressings.

Relationships to remember

1 dm = 0.1 m
1 m = 10 dm

1 cm = 0.01 m
1 m = 100 cm

1 mm = 0.001 m
1 m = 1000 mm

EXAMPLE 4.1

Here are some examples of these abbreviations in use.

- A roll of hypoallergenic surgical tape is 12.5 mm in width and 10 m in length.
- The compression bandaging required by an elderly female patient for the treatment of a venous leg ulcer is 10 cm wide and has a stretched length of 4.7 m.
- The average height for an adult in the UK is 163.7 cm for women and 176.8 cm for men.
- In the first year of their life a child's head grows by about 1 dm in circumference.
- The body lengths of most newborn babies in the UK lie within the range 45 to 56 cm.

How are lengths converted between these different units?

We introduced the *decimetre* above because it helps us to see how these metric units of length relate to the way the number system works: the units, tenths, hundredths and thousandths in a decimal number (see Chapter 1) can be interpreted as metres, decimetres, centimetres and millimetres in a length. Consider for example, the length 2.345 metres. The 2 in the units position represents 2 metres, of course. The 3 in the tenths position represents 3 tenths of a metre, which is 3 decimetres. The 4 in the hundredths position represents 4 hundredths of a metre, which is 4 centimetres. And the 5 in the thousandths position represents 5 thousandths of a metre, which is 5 millimetres. So, we have this very simple expansion: 2.345 m = 2 m + 3 dm + 4 cm + 5 mm.

EXAMPLE 4.2

(a) In the same way, 0.435 metres can be expanded like this:

0.435 m = 0 m + 4 dm + 3 cm + 5 mm (= 4 dm + 3 cm + 5 mm).

(b) Similarly, 0.058 m = 0 m + 0 dm + 5 cm + 8 mm (= 5 cm + 8 mm)

To change a measurement of length between metres, decimetres, centimetres, and millimetres, we can apply these two principles:

A To convert from metres to decimetres, or from decimetres to centimetres, or from centimetres to millimetres, we *multiply* by 10.

B To convert from millimetres to centimetres, or from centimetres to decimetres, or from decimetres to metres, we *divide* by 10.

EXAMPLE 4.3

(a) Convert a length of 1.34 metres to decimetres. There are 10 decimetres in a metre, so we must multiply by 10. Moving the decimal point one place to the right, we get 1.34 m = 13.4 dm.

(b) Convert a length of 0.4 centimetres to millimetres. There are 10 millimetres in a centimetre, so we must multiply by 10. Moving the decimal point one place to the right, we get 0.4 cm = 4 mm.

EXAMPLE 4.4

(a) Convert a length of 2.5 millimetres to centimetres. Now we must divide by 10. Moving the decimal point one place to the left, we then get 2.5 mm = 0.25 cm.

(b) Convert a length of 75 centimetres to decimetres. Again we must divide by 10. Moving the decimal point one place to the left, we get 75 cm = 7.5 dm.

Metres to centimetres

Multiply by 100:
  1.65 m = 165 cm
  0.875 m = 87.5 cm

Centimetres to metres

Divide by 100:
  58 cm = 0.58 m
  1250 cm = 12.50 m

Changing between metres and centimetres is common in recording the heights of patients, for example. Because there are 100 centimetres in a metre, this is done by multiplication or division by 100. It is helpful to note that the relationship between metres and centimetres is exactly the same as the familiar relationship in money between pounds and pence.

EXAMPLE 4.5

(a) Change 1.56 m to centimetres. Think: £1.56 = 156 p, so 1.56 m = 156 cm.

(b) Change 75 cm to metres. Think: 75 p = £0.75, so 75 cm = 0.75 m.

In a similar way, because there are 1000 millimetres in a metre, changing between metres and millimetres will require multiplication or division by 1000. This means shifting the decimal point three places.

Metres to millimetres	Millimetres to metres
Multiply by 1000:	Divide by 1000:
1.65 m = 1650 mm	67 mm = 0.067 m
0.875 m = 875 mm	1250 mm = 1.250 m
	(= 1.25 m)

EXAMPLE 4.6

(a) Convert a height of 1.54 metres to millimetres. Because there are 1000 millimetres in a metre we must multiply the 1.54 by 1000. This requires shifting the decimal point three places to the right, which gives us 1.54 m = 1540 mm.

(b) Convert a length of 750 mm to metres. We must divide by 1000, which involves shifting the decimal point three places to the left. This gives us 750 mm = 0.750 m. This may be written as 0.75 m.

What about reading lengths and heights from measuring scales?

There are various kinds of digital devices available for measuring height, for which the healthcare practitioner has only to set up the device and read off the measurement from a digital display. But often a healthcare practitioner will need to read accurately from a linear scale, such as on a tape measure or any kind of non-digital device for measuring the length/height of an infant or the height of a child or adult. A *stadiometer,* for example, is a device for measuring the height of a patient who is able to stand. This consists of a vertical ruler with a sliding horizontal rod or paddle that is adjusted to rest on the top of the head. The height of the patient is read off from the portion of the scale revealed in a window, as shown in Figure 4.2. This shows the reading from a stadiometer used to measure the height of a 3-year-old child. Each small interval between the centimetre marks is a millimetre (a tenth of a centimetre). The pointer indicates that this height is six millimetres above 91 cm, so the height is read off as 91.6 cm, or 916 mm. In Chapter 8, we explain that this is the height 'to the nearest tenth of a centimetre' or 'to the nearest millimetre'.

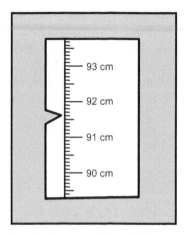

Figure 4.2 The height of a 3-year-old child shown in a stadiometer window

4.1   Write this as a single measurement in metres: 2 m + 9 cm + 4 mm.

4.2   Convert:

(a) 1.4 m to millimetres   (b) 105 cm to metres

(c) 0.7 cm to millimetres   (d) 75 mm to metres

4.3   Which of the following is (a) the longest length? (b) the shortest length?

49.5 cm, 0.459 m, 4059 mm, 5 dm?

4.4   The length of a baby two weeks after birth is measured and found to lie half-way between 46 and 47 centimetres. What would this length be in centimetres? In millimetres?

4.5   Read off the height indicated by the pointer in the window in Figure 4.3, in centimetres. What would this be in metres?

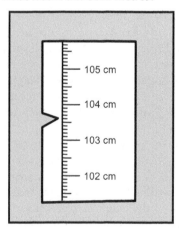

Figure 4.3   What is the height indicated by the pointer?
(check-up question 4.5)

4.6   A girl aged 12 years has a height of 1.39 m. In three months she grows by 1 cm. What is her new height in metres?

UNITS OF
LIQUID VOLUME 5

OBJECTIVES

In a practical healthcare context the practitioner should be able to:

- make reasonable estimates of capacities of containers in litres or millilitres
- recall the relationship between litres and millilitres
- use correctly the terminology, conventions and abbreviations for recording liquid volume and capacity measured in litres and millilitres
- convert measurements of capacity and liquid volume between litres and millilitres

SPOT THE ERRORS

Identify any obvious errors in the following ten statements.

1 The standard units for measuring liquid volume are the litre (l) and the millilitre (ml).

2 One litre of a liquid is the same volume as 100 millilitres (100 ml).

3 An adult male's total urine output for a period of 24 hours is recorded as 950 ml, which is less than a litre.

4 A standard wine bottle holds 7.5 decilitres of wine.

5 A standard medicine spoon holds up to 5 Ml of liquid.

6 A 500-ml bottle of mouthwash is equivalent to half a litre.

7 A millilitre is one thousandth of a litre, which is 0.001 litres.

8 A dose of 1170 litres is the same as 1.170 millilitres.

9 A volume of 0.06 litres expressed in millilitres is 60 ml.

10 An infusion pump is set at 10 ml per hour in order to deliver a total volume of 0.4 litres of a preparation over 4 hours.

Are the errors you have spotted potentially serious in medical health practice?

(errors identified on page 60)

What are litres and millilitres?

Litres and millilitres are the standard units used for measuring liquid volume and capacity. The volume of something is the amount of three-dimensional space it takes up. Volumes of solids are usually measured in units such as the *cubic metre* (the volume of a cube with side of length 1 metre) or the *cubic centimetre* (the volume of a cube of side 1 centimetre). But it has become standard practice to measure liquid volume in units called litres and millilitres, even though these are not officially SI units (see Chapter 4). A litre is actually the volume of water that weighs the same as 1 kilogram (see Chapter 6). This is the same volume as 1000 cubic centimetres – imagine a cube of side 10 cm. And a millilitre is the same volume as 1 cubic centimetre.

The word *capacity* refers to containers. The capacity of a container is the maximum volume of liquid that it can hold. Capacity is therefore also measured in litres and millilitres. For example, a syringe might have a capacity of 10 millilitres, meaning that it can be used to draw up to 10 millilitres of liquid. We should note that in practice there is a distinction between the *nominal capacity*, which is the volume the container is intended to hold, and the *brimful capacity*, which is what it could hold if it were to be filled absolutely to the brim. In the case of the 10-millilitres syringe, for example, 10 millilitres is the nominal capacity, which should not normally be exceeded – in fact the scale marked on such a syringe will go up to 10 millilitres and no further. Similarly, a 1-litre measuring jug will actually hold a little more than a litre if filled to the brim, but the scale will go only up to 1000 millilitres.

The prefix *milli*, as we noted in Chapter 4, means 'a thousandth', so a millilitre is one thousandth of a litre. This means, of course that a litre is one thousand millilitres.

Remember then: 1 litre = 1000 millilitres and 1 millilitre = 0.001 litres.

Our confidence in handling any units of measurement is boosted by having a good sense of their approximate magnitude and making use of reference items. A litre is easy to imagine because so many liquid products are purchased in litre containers: look out for a 1-litre carton of fruit juice or milk, for example. Remember also that a standard medicine spoon will hold up to 5 millilitres of medicine: this is a very handy reference item.

> **Some reference items for litres and millilitres**
>
> - The most common cartons of fruit juice hold 1 litre.
> - A normal young adult could have a bladder capacity of up to about half a litre (500 millilitres).
> - A standard size for a can of soft drink is 330 millilitres (about a third of a litre).
> - A standard medicine spoon can hold up to 5 millilitres.
> - A millilitre is the same volume as a cube of side 1 cm.

What are the standard abbreviations for these units of liquid volume?

The abbreviation for the litre is the single letter 'l' (el). This is a problem, because when hand-written or printed in some fonts it looks like the numeral 1 (one). Our advice is to write the words *litre* and *litres* in full to avoid confusion. The correct abbreviation for

> **Litres and millilitres**
>
> 1 litre = 1000 ml
> 1 ml = 0.001 litres

ERRORS IDENTIFIED

The obvious errors are Statements 2, 5, 8 and 10.

Statement 2

One litre is 1000 millilitres (1000 ml), not 100 millilitres. Note that Statement 7 is correct: a millilitre is one *thousandth* of a litre. As we saw in Chapter 4, the prefix *milli* means 'one thousandth'. So, just as a metre is 1000 millimetres, so a litre is one thousand millilitres. Knowing and using accurately the relationship between litres and millilitres is fundamental to healthcare practice, and it would be seriously worrying if a practitioner thought that 100 ml was the same as a litre.

Statement 5

The spoon will hold up to *5 millilitres* of a liquid. The abbreviation for *millilitre* is *ml*, not *Ml*. A lower case *m* is used as the abbreviation for *milli* (one thousandth), not an upper case *M* (which is the abbreviation for 'mega', meaning a million!). This error is sloppy and looks unprofessional.

Statement 8

The units of liquid volume are the wrong way round in this statement. It should read: a volume of 1170 millilitres is 1.170 litre. If you did not spot this error then take this as a warning about how we can all overlook the most glaring errors when we read things in a hurry. In practice it is unlikely that anyone would attempt to administer a dose of 1170 litres of a preparation, since this would weigh more than a ton!

Statement 10

In 4 hours an infusion pump set at 10 ml per hour will deliver 40 ml. This is 0.04 litres, not 0.4 litres (which would be 400 ml). To deliver 400 ml in 4 hours the pump should be set at 100 ml per hour. This is potentially a serious error in a healthcare context. In a paediatric or an intensive care unit, for example, delivering only a tenth of what is required may have serious clinical implications for a patient's well-being. We explain calculations involving infusion rates and the use of 'per' in Chapter 12.

(now continue reading from page 59)

millilitres, which we shall use, is 'ml'. However, in healthcare contexts, it is not unusual to see a capital L used for litre and mL for millilitre.

EXAMPLE 5.1

Here are some examples of these units in use.

- Examples of common capacities for syringes are 1 ml, 2 ml, 5 ml, 10 ml, 20 ml and 50 ml.
- A 1-ml syringe would be used to draw a volume up to and including 1 ml, for example, 0.6 ml.
- One manufacturer's range of P.E.T. (polyethylene terephthalate) medicine bottles includes bottles with nominal capacities of 60 ml, 70 ml, 100 ml, 125 ml, 150 ml, 250 ml, 300 ml, 500 ml (0.5 litres) and 1 litre.
- The brimful capacity of a P.E.T. bottle with nominal capacity of 60 ml is 67 ml, and that of the 500-ml bottle is 543 ml.
- For a particular patient, a patient-controlled analgesia infusion pump is programmed to deliver a single bolus dose of 0.5 ml (half a millilitre) of a morphine preparation when required.
- Intravenous metronidazole is supplied in pre-prepared bags each containing a volume of 100 ml. A batch of 10 of these bags would contain altogether 1 litre (1000 ml) of the preparation.

A common volume of fluid used in healthcare practice is 100 ml. We shall see in Chapter 13, for example, that concentrations are often expressed as the amount of a substance dissolved in 100 ml. A volume of 100 ml is a tenth of a litre (0.1 litres), which is therefore a *decilitre*. So a concentration of so much in 100 ml is often expressed in terms of so much in a decilitre. The correct abbreviation for decilitre is dl, but dL is also used extensively in practice.

Note for wine drinkers: a standard bottle of wine provides you with 750 ml of wine. The bottle will sometimes be labelled 0.75 litres. We have also seen bottles labelled 7.5 dl (7.5 decilitres) or 75 cl (75 centilitres): a *centilitre* is a hundredth of a litre (1 cl = 0.01 litres = 10 ml). A unit of alcohol, used for making recommendations about levels of alcohol consumption, is defined in the UK as 10 ml. This is what you would get in 80 ml of wine (12.5% strength). We recommend the red.

How are volumes converted between these different units?

In a healthcare context you will come across quantities of liquid recorded sometimes in litres and sometimes in millilitres. Practitioners should be able to convert between these units instantly, without any difficulty. So, for example, a bottle marked as containing

250 ml is recognized as containing 0.25 litres; and liquid to a level of 0.4 litres in a litre measuring jug is understood to indicate a volume of 400 millilitres.

The mathematical principles for conversion between litres and millilitres are illustrated in Figure 5.1.

A To convert from litres to millilitres we *multiply* by 1000.

B To convert from millilitres to litres we *divide* by a thousand.

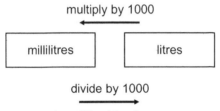

Figure 5.1   Converting units of liquid volume

EXAMPLE 5.2

(a) Convert 1.25 litres to millilitres. We must multiply by 1000. (See Figure 5.1.) It helps us here to make sure that there are at least three digits after the decimal point by thinking of 1.25 litres as 1.250 litres. Then, moving the decimal point three places to the right, we get 1.250 litres = 1250 ml.

(b) Convert 0.075 litres to millilitres. We must multiply by 1000. Moving the decimal point three places to the right, we get 0.075 litres = 75 ml.

EXAMPLE 5.3

(a) Convert 12.5 ml to litres. Now we must divide by 1000. (See Figure 5.1.) Moving the decimal point three places to the left, we get 12.5 ml = 0.0125 litres. Note the need for a zero as a place-holder in the tenths position and an additional leading zero in front of the decimal point.

(b) Convert 1170 ml to litres. Again we must divide by 1000. Moving the decimal point three places to the left, we get 1170 ml = 1.170 litres. This may be written as 1.17 litres.

5.1   Match each of the items listed below with the most likely capacity.

A wall-mounted hand sanitizer dispenser   150 ml

A vial of the antibiotic gentamicin   5.7 litres

A small bottle of water   2 ml

A syringe for a blood sample sufficient for a range of tests   0.8 litres

A hospital cleaner's bucket   20 ml

A small glass of wine   250 ml

5.2   Convert:

(a) 1.25 litres to ml   (b) 1400 ml to litres

(c) 0.05 litres to ml   (d) 6 ml to litres

5.3   Which of the following is (a) the largest volume? (b) the smallest volume?

500 ml, 0.525 litres, 0.065 litres, 0.53 litres, 99 ml.

5.4   A neonate requires an intramuscular injection of 0.1 ml of a phytomenadione preparation. From the syringes listed in Example 5.1 earlier in the chapter, what size syringe would be used to draw this volume of the preparation?

5.5   An infusion pump is set to deliver 20 ml of heparin infusion each hour. What volume is delivered in 8 hours? Give the answer:

(a) in millilitres   (b) in litres

5.6   A patient requires 0.6 litres of fluid over 5 hours using an infusion pump.

(a) How many millilitres are delivered in an hour?

(b) Convert the answer to (a) to litres.

5.7   A hospital patient's urine output is measured on five occasions during a day, as 250 ml, 375 ml, 400 ml, 180 ml and 245 ml. What is the total of these measurements? Give the answer:

(a) in millilitres   (b) in litres

UNITS OF WEIGHT

6

OBJECTIVES

In a practical healthcare context the practitioner should be able to:

- make reasonable estimates of weights in kilograms and grams and have a sense of the magnitude of a milligram and a microgram
- recall the relationships between kilograms, grams, milligrams and micrograms
- use correctly the terminology, conventions and abbreviations for recording weight measured in kilograms, grams, milligrams and micrograms
- convert measurements of weight between grams and milligrams, and between milligrams and micrograms

SPOT THE ERRORS

Identify any obvious errors in the following ten statements.

1 A male adult patient's weight is recorded as 745 kg.

2 A newborn baby's weight is recorded as 3.6 kg, which is 3600 g.

3 A 1-litre bottle will hold 1 kg of water.

4 A standard medicine spoon holds up to 5 grams of water.

5 A 500-mg tablet is equivalent to half a gram.

6 A microgram is a millionth of a gram.

7 A dose of 25 micrograms is written as 25 mg.

8 A weight of 5 milligrams is equal to 0.005 g.

9 A dose of 150 mg of an antibiotic given three times daily is 4.5 g per day.

10 A concentration of 0.5 milligrams of a substance per litre is the same as 500 micrograms per litre.

Are the errors you have spotted potentially serious in medical health practice?

(errors identified over the page)

ERRORS IDENTIFIED

The obvious errors are Statements 1, 7 and 9.

Statement 1

A body weight of 745 kg would be nearly three-quarters of a tonne. No human being has ever been recorded as weighing this much! It is likely that a fairly normal weight of 74.5 kg has been wrongly recorded in this statement. This error would be embarrassing for the practitioner who makes it and has the potential to be serious if a drug dosage is required to be calculated based on a patient's weight. However, knowing the medication involved and making a reasonable estimate of the dosage required as part of the calculation should alert the practitioner to the recording error.

Statement 7

The abbreviation *mg* stands for *milligram*, not *microgram*. The simple fact that *milli* and *micro* begin with the same letter can be the cause of potential confusion. So a dose of 25 *milligrams* would be written as 25 mg. We discuss abbreviations for micrograms below. Clearly, this is potentially a serious error in the context of healthcare practice, since a dose of 25 milligrams would be 1000 times a dose of 25 micrograms. As an example, consider the implications for a patient who is given 62.5 milligrams of digoxin instead of a typical dose of 62.5 micrograms.

Statement 9

Multiplying 150 by three gives 450. So three doses of 150 mg (milligrams) are equivalent to 450 mg. In grams this is 0.450 g per day. A total of 4.5 g per day would be 4500 mg, which is ten times larger. We discuss conversions between grams and milligrams below. A ten-times dosage error is a common cause of patient harm. This is potentially a more serious error than in Statement 7, because in practice a dose 1000 times too large is more likely to be spotted before being administered than one that is 10 times too large or too small.

What are kilograms, grams, milligrams and micrograms?

Kilograms, grams, milligrams and micrograms are the standard and most common units used for measuring weight in a healthcare context. Working from left to right, each unit is equivalent to a thousand of the next one. A kilogram is 1000 grams, a gram is 1000 milligrams, and a milligram is 1000 micrograms.

This means, therefore, that, working from right to the left, each unit is one thousandth (0.001) of the previous one. A microgram is 0.001 of a milligram, a milligram is 0.001 of a gram, and a gram is 0.001 of a kilogram. Note the correct spelling of the word *gram* (not *gramme*).

Our confidence in handling any units of measurement is boosted by having a good sense of their approximate magnitude. A kilogram is the easiest to relate to because that is the weight of a litre of water. So, think of a litre carton of fruit juice and you've got approximately a kilogram. If you prefer it, think of a standard bottle of wine, which, including the bottle, will also weigh something of the order of one kilogram.

As we noted in Chapter 4, the prefix *kilo* means 'a thousand'; so, for example, a kilometre is 1000 metres and a kilowatt is 1000 watts – and a kilogram is 1000 grams.

So, what would weigh about one gram? It would be something that you would hardly notice if someone put it in your outstretched hand while your eyes were closed. Think of a piece of paper about the size of a postcard: that would be about one gram in weight.

We met the prefix *milli*, meaning 'one thousandth' in the millimetre (one thousandth of a metre) and the millilitre (one thousandth of a litre) in previous chapters. In the same way a milligram is one thousandth of a gram. So, cut the one-gram piece of paper into 1000 tiny pieces and each of them would weigh about a milligram. If you cut out one of the letters in this sentence, the piece of paper would weigh something of the order of 1 milligram! You would certainly not be aware of the weight of an object weighing a milligram if it were placed in your hand.

And since a microgram is one thousandth of a milligram, we're talking about a very tiny weight now. The prefix *micro* means one millionth, so there are one million micrograms in a gram. A piece of paper weighing 1 microgram would be smaller than the full stop at the end of this sentence.

Note for scientific purists: kilograms, grams, milligrams and micrograms are actually units of mass, not weight, a subtle distinction we will not attempt to explain here. In this book we use the word *weight* as it is commonly used in most medical contexts as a synonym for *mass*. A familiar healthcare context in which the correct word *mass* is used is the *body-mass index* (explained in Chapter 14). The weight of an object is

Some reference items for kilograms and grams

- A typical international rugby centre might weigh around 100 kg.
- A typical male professional jockey might weigh around 50 kg.
- Typical weights of newborn babies are 3 to 4 kilograms.
- A litre of water weighs a kilogram.
- An individual packet of crisps weighs about 30 grams.
- A small (5-ml) medicine spoon holds up to 5 grams of water.

strictly speaking the force of gravity acting on the object and would therefore be measured in units of force, namely, *newtons*.

What are the standard abbreviations for these units of weight?

Relationships to remember

1 kg = 1000 g
1 g = 0.001 kg

1 mg = 0.001 g
1 g = 1000 mg

1 microgram = 0.001 mg
1 mg = 1000 micrograms

In previous chapters we have introduced the abbreviations for the prefixes *deci* (d), *centi* (c) and *milli* (m). In the context of weight the only one of these usually required is that for *milli*: the milligram is abbreviated to mg. But for measurements of weight we need two further abbreviations. The symbol for *kilo* (a thousand) is k (a lower case k, not an upper case K). The symbol for *micro* (a millionth) is the Greek letter μ (mu). So we have kg, g, mg and μg as the symbols for kilogram, gram, milligram and microgram, respectively.

In a healthcare context the abbreviation mcg is often used for microgram. However, it is good practice for 'micrograms' to be written in full as this reduces the risk of an error. It is recommended that the abbreviation μg should not be used in practice, even though it is strictly correct, as this can easily be mistaken for 'mg' – particularly when handwritten – and lead to a serious dosing error.

EXAMPLE 6.1

Here are some examples of these abbreviations in use.

- A woman with obesity weighs 123 kg (123 kilograms).
- A nurse records a patient's faecal output as 140 g (140 grams).
- A tablet of the beta-blocker atenolol contains 25 mg (25 milligrams) of the drug.
- An inhaler delivers a dose of 200 micrograms of the steroid beclometasone.
- A man with atrial fibrillation is prescribed 62.5 micrograms of digoxin daily.

How are weights converted between these different units?

There are two simple principles to grasp here, illustrated in Figure 6.1:

A To convert from kilograms to grams, or from grams to milligrams, or from milligrams to micrograms, we *multiply* by 1000.

B To convert from micrograms to milligrams, or from milligrams to grams, or from grams to kilograms, we *divide* by 1000.

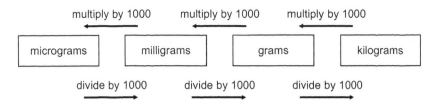

Figure 6.1   Converting units of weight

EXAMPLE 6.2

(See Figure 6.1.)

(a) Convert 1.34 kilograms to grams. We must multiply by 1000. It helps us to make sure that there are at least three digits after the decimal point by thinking of 1.34 kg as 1.340 kg. Then, shifting the decimal point three places to the right, we get 1.340 kg = 1340 g.

(b) Convert 0.4 milligrams to micrograms. We must multiply by 1000. Again, it helps us to make sure that there are at least three digits after the decimal point by thinking of 0.4 mg as 0.400 mg. Then, shifting the decimal point three places to the right, we get 0.400 mg = 400 micrograms.

(c) Convert 0.075 grams to milligrams. We must multiply by 1000. Shifting the decimal point three places to the right, we get 0.075 g = 75 mg.

EXAMPLE 6.3

(See Figure 6.1.)

(a) Convert 2.5 milligrams to grams. Now we must divide by 1000. Shifting the decimal point three places to the left, we get 2.5 mg = 0.0025 g. Note the zeros required as place-holders in the first two places after the decimal point and the additional leading zero placed in front of the decimal point.

(b) Convert 2560 grams to kilograms. Again we must divide by 1000. Shifting the decimal point three places to the left we get 2560 g = 2.560 kg. This may be written as 2.56 kg.

(c) Convert 75 micrograms to milligrams. We must divide by 1000. Shifting the decimal point three places to the left, we get 75 micrograms = 0.075 milligrams. Again note the zero required as a place-holder in the tenths position and the additional leading zero in front of the decimal point.

In what situations are weights converted between these different units?

Below are four examples of situations in which weights might sometimes be converted from one unit to another. First, when the result of a calculation involving units of weight is an answer greater than 1000 units.

EXAMPLE 6.4

You calculate the total daily dose of a drug given in four equally-divided doses of 300 milligrams. Now, $300 \times 4 = 1200$, so the result is 1200 mg. It may be clearer to record this as 1.2 g.

Second, when the result of a calculation involving units of weight is an answer less than 1 unit.

EXAMPLE 6.5

A 14-year-old's daily dosage of penicillin V is 2.0 g. This is to be administered in four equal doses, one every 6 hours. The calculation required is $2.0 \div 4$, which equals 0.5. So each dose should be 0.5 g. It may be more convenient to record this as 500 mg.

Third, when you have to do any calculation involving measurements of weight that are given in different units.

EXAMPLE 6.6

You have to find how many doses of 50 milligrams there are in a total weight of 2 grams. You cannot divide the 2 g by the 50 mg as they stand, because they are in different units. So you could convert the 2 g to 2000 mg. Then you can divide 2000 by 50 to calculate the number of doses. (The answer is 40.)

Fourth, to simplify a calculation involving decimals.

EXAMPLE 6.7

A patient requires 1.75 g of amoxicillin per day, to be administered in two equal doses every 12 hours. To find the individual dose you would need to divide 1.75 g by 2. Some practitioners may be more confident with this calculation if they convert the 1.75 g to 1750 mg. There are now no decimal numbers involved in the calculation: $1750 \div 2 = 875$. So the individual dose is 875 mg (or 0.875 g). This idea is developed in Chapter 9 where we look in more detail at calculations involving decimal numbers.

6.1 Convert:

   (a) 1.25 mg to micrograms   (b) 7250 grams to kilograms

6.2 Which of the following is (a) the largest dose? (b) the smallest dose?

   500 mg, 0.275 g, 5000 micrograms, 0.6 g, 6 mg.

6.3 A child's daily dosage of erythromycin is 1.5 g, to be administered in four equal doses, one every 6 hours. What is the dose required every 6 hours,

   (a) in milligrams?   (b) in grams?

6.4 How many 50-mg doses of Drug A would give a total dosage of 4 grams?

6.5 A dosage of 5 mg of Drug B for each kilogram of a person's weight is required. What is the correct dosage for an adult weighing 70 kg,

   (a) in milligrams?   (b) in grams?

HAVE A CHECK-UP

USING A
CALCULATOR

7

OBJECTIVES

In a practical healthcare context the practitioner should be able to:

- use both basic and scientific calculators to perform calculations, showing awareness of their different operating systems
- enter calculations accurately onto a calculator and interpret the answer displayed
- identify the calculation or sequence of calculations to be entered on a calculator in a range of situations
- check results and recognize when a calculator answer is clearly incorrect because of an error in entering data
- use the memory facility on a calculator to store and retrieve numbers arising in calculations

SPOT THE ERRORS

Identify any obvious errors in the use of calculators in the following seven statements.

1   A practitioner who needs to multiply the sum of 2.8 and 8.4 by 6.2 enters '2.8 + 8.4 × 6.2 =' onto a scientific calculator and gets the result 54.88.

2   The prescribed dosage of darbepoetin alpha is 2.25 micrograms per kg of a child's weight; to calculate the dosage in micrograms for a child weighing 18.9 kg a nurse enters '18.9 × 2.25 =' onto a calculator and gets the result 42.525.

3   To find the infusion rate in millilitres per hour required if 1500 ml is to be infused over a 24-hour period a practitioner enters onto a calculator '1500 ÷ 24 =' and gets the result 62.5.

4   To divide a total of 6 grams of a drug into 8 doses, a practitioner enters '6 ÷ 8 =' onto a calculator, reads off the result 0.75 and concludes that each dose should be 75 milligrams.

5   A patient's body surface area is estimated to be 1.95 square metres; the dosage for a drug is 120 mg per square metre of body surface area. On a calculator '120 × 1.95 =' is entered to calculate the dosage; the result displayed is 234, which indicates 234 mg, or 0.234 g.

6   To check that the result 2.625 for the calculation 47.25 ÷ 18 is correct, a practitioner uses the calculator to multiply the 2.625 by 18, expecting to get the result 47.25.

7   The following key sequence on a calculator will generate the result 70: MC, 17, +, 18, =, M+, 20, -, 18, =, ×, MR, =
    (MC = 'memory clear', M+ = add to memory, MR = memory recall)

Are the errors you have spotted potentially serious in medical health practice?

(errors identified over the page)

ERRORS IDENTIFIED

The obvious errors are in Statements 1 and 4.

Statement 1

It should be obvious that there must be an error here, because 2.8 + 8.4 is clearly greater than 10, which when multiplied by a number greater than 6 must give an answer greater than 60. The error has occurred because a scientific calculator gives precedence to multiplication over addition. It does not just do the operations in the order in which they are entered. So for the key sequence '2.8 + 8.4 × 6.2 =' the calculator will not add the 2.8 and the 8.4 until it has first identified what follows the 8.4. When '× 6.2 =' is entered it multiplies the 8.4 by the 6.2, before adding the result of this to the 2.8. Using brackets to indicate what gets done first, this calculator has found 2.8 + (8.4 × 6.2), whereas what was required was (2.8 + 8.4) × 6.2. We explain different calculator operating systems and brackets below. This is a potentially serious error, because it indicates that the practitioner could easily enter the wrong key sequence for an important calculation onto their calculator. This also suggests that the practitioner is not routinely checking calculator results to ensure that they are reasonable.

Statement 4

The error here is that the 0.75 displayed represents 0.75 g, which is 750 mg, not 75 mg as stated. We explain below the importance of remembering that calculators do not display 'trailing zeros'. For example, a calculator result of 0.180 litres (180 ml) will be displayed as 0.18. This would represent not 18 ml, but 180 ml. This is clearly a potentially serious error, particularly if this led to a dosage that is only a tenth of what is required.

What is the difference between a basic calculator and a scientific calculator?

When we refer to a *basic calculator* we are talking about an electronic calculator with keys for four basic operations: addition, subtraction, multiplication and division, and not much more, as shown in Figure 7.1(a). The key labelled *CE* (clear entry) is pressed to clear whatever is on display.

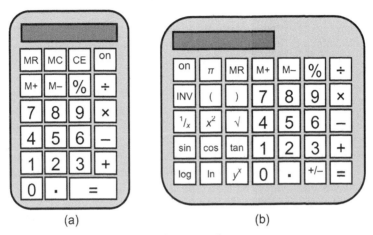

(a)   (b)

Figure 7.1   Calculators: (a) basic, (b) scientific

A basic calculator will probably have a number of other keys, such as M+, M−, MC, MR, which are for accessing the memory facility of the calculator: these are explained later in this chapter. Some basic calculators may also have keys for calculating a percentage (%) and some may have a key for finding a square root (√). The use of the percentage key on a calculator is explained in Chapter 13; square roots are used in calculations of body weight in Chapter 14.

You can easily recognize what we are calling a *scientific calculator* because it will have keys for brackets as well as for other mathematical functions such as sines and cosines, logarithms and exponential functions. All these functions are beyond the scope of this book and are unlikely to be needed in practical healthcare contexts. A scientific calculator may look something like Figure 7.1(b).

Practitioners may have access to either of these two kinds of calculator and must therefore be aware of the essential distinction between them: the different ways in which they deal with a sequence of steps in calculations. Most basic calculators have a 'non-algebraic' operating system for calculations. This just means that they deal with each step of a calculation in the order in which the steps are entered. Here's a really easy example to illustrate this.

EXAMPLE 7.1

A patient is prescribed one tablet four times daily for 12 days, followed by one tablet twice daily for the next 16 days. What is the correct number of tablets that the patient requires for the first 28 days of treatment? That's 12 days on 4 tablets and 16 days on 2 tablets. The calculation required therefore is 12 × 4 + 16 × 2.

Basic and scientific calculators: spot the difference!

A basic calculator deals with calculations in the order in which they are entered. For example:
'4 + 2 × 7 =' gives the result 42.
A scientific calculator gives precedence to multiplication and division over addition and subtraction, unless brackets are used. For example:
'4 + 2 × 7 =' gives the result 18;
'(4 + 2) × 7 =' gives the result 42.

Now we know that most readers could do this mentally while standing on their head and playing the Beethoven Violin Concerto. But it will be instructive to look at how we might do this calculation on a calculator. If you have access to a calculator, switch it on and press this sequence of keys: 12 × 4 + 16 × 2 =. If you get the (incorrect) answer 128, then the calculator you are using is what we are calling a basic calculator. It has a *non-algebraic* operating system. It has done the operations in the order they were entered: it multiplied 12 by 4, added 16 to the result and then multiplied this answer by 2.

If, however, you get the (correct) answer 80, then your calculator is what we are calling a scientific calculator. It has an *algebraic* operating system. The calculator has decided to do the multiplications of 12 by 4 and 16 by 2 before it deals with the addition.

If you have not yet done so, now would be a good time to access the calculators you have on devices such as computers and mobile telephones and check whether or not they use an algebraic operating system. To do this, press this sequence of keys: '4 + 2 × 7 ='. If you get the result 42, the calculator is a basic one and does not have an algebraic operating system. If, however, you get the answer 18, it does have an algebraic operating system, the system used by scientific calculators.

Evidently, it is important to be clear about which operating system your calculator uses for calculations – otherwise it may give you the answer to a different calculation from the one you thought you were doing! Imagine this scenario.

EXAMPLE 7.2

A grandmother telephones a practice nurse to report that her 4-year-old grandson has become unwell with a fever and that he has a temperature of 101 degrees. The nurse realizes this must be a Fahrenheit temperature and remembers that you can convert it to Celsius by subtracting 32 and dividing by 1.8. Without a conversion chart to hand, the nurse picks up a nearby calculator and presses this sequence of keys: '101 – 32 ÷ 1.8 ='. The result displayed is: 83.222222. Is this really the child's temperature in degrees Celsius? What kind of calculator has the nurse picked up?

The nurse wanted to subtract 32 from 101 first and then divide by 1.8. The calculator has not done the calculations in the order they were entered. Instead it has done the division of 32 by 1.8 first and then subtracted the answer to this from 101. This indicates that the nurse is using a scientific calculator with an algebraic operating system. It has given precedence to the division over the subtraction. Let's hope that the story continues as below!

EXAMPLE 7.2 (CONTINUED)

The nurse realized that the child's temperature could not possibly be 83.2 degrees Celsius and that the calculator is not the usual basic one used in the practice but a scientific one. The nurse then found a basic calculator and entered the same sequence of keys ('101 − 32 ÷ 1.8 =') and got the correct answer for converting 101 degrees Fahrenheit to degrees Celsius: 38.333333. The nurse rounded this to 38.3 degrees Celsius (see Chapter 8 for rounding) and arranged for the boy to come to the practice for a review.

To deal with this and other calculations correctly on a scientific calculator we have to be alert to the principles of *precedence of operators* and how *brackets* are used in calculations.

Can you explain precedence of operators and brackets?

Justifiably, the reader may have been confused in the previous section by arithmetical statements like '4 + 2 × 7'. How do we know whether this means 'four add 2 and then multiply the answer by 7' or 'add 4 to what you get by multiplying 2 by 7'? Well, in practice, it is the context that gave rise to the calculation that makes it clear to us what is meant. In Example 7.1 above the context makes it clear that '12 × 4 + 16 × 2' means that we have to multiply 12 by 4 and multiply 16 by 2 and then add the two products. A problem would occur only if a practitioner were to enter the calculation as written down onto a calculator without thinking about what the calculation means and without checking what kind of calculator they were using.

Precedence of operators

Unless the context that gives rise to a calculation indicates something different:

- do any calculations inside brackets first
- then do any multiplications and divisions
- then do any additions and subtractions

When we don't know the context and just see arithmetical statements like these written down baldly, they can be ambiguous. To avoid this mathematicians have the principle of *precedence of operators*. This is simply that in a potentially ambiguous statement of a calculation, it is assumed that any multiplications or divisions will be done first, taking precedence over addition and subtraction.

So if we are presented with '4 + 2 × 7', without any contextual information, we assume that this means that we should do the multiplication first, and that the result of the calculation is therefore 18, not 42.

The principle of precedence of operators always applies without exception in algebraic expressions, as we shall explain in Chapter 14. Also, anyone who enters formulas into computer spreadsheets should be aware that these invariably use the principle of precedence of operators.

Brackets

Use brackets generously when writing down calculations using more than one operation to avoid any ambiguity about what should be done first.

To avoid ambiguity we can also use *brackets* to indicate which calculations should be done first. Operations inside brackets always take precedence over anything else. So, in the example above of the nurse converting a child's temperature to degrees Celsius, the calculation would best be written as (101 – 32) ÷ 1.8, making it absolutely clear that the 32 has to be subtracted from the 101 first.

We recommend using brackets quite generously when writing down calculations, whenever there is any possibility of ambiguity, even when strictly they are not necessary. So, for example, although '12 × 4 + 16 × 2' is not strictly ambiguous, because of the precedence of operators principle, there is no room for getting the order of calculations wrong if we stick in some brackets, like this: (12 × 4) + (16 × 2).

So when we say that scientific calculators have an algebraic operating system, we mean that they give precedence to multiplication and division over addition and subtraction. Scientific calculators also have keys for entering brackets, so the nurse in our temperature example could enter the calculations required on a scientific calculator by pressing this whole sequence of keys, including the keys for opening and closing brackets: (101 – 32) ÷ 1.8 =.

Basic calculators do not have keys for brackets. So, if we needed to calculate, for example, (47.5 × 4) – (62.5 × 3), we would either have to write down some of the intermediate results, or use the memory facility if the calculator has one.

How do you use the memory keys on a basic calculator?

Using the memory facility

Use the memory facility on a basic calculator to store and access intermediate results. *MC* sets the memory to zero *M+* adds what is displayed to the memory *M–* subtracts what is displayed from the memory *MR* displays the number currently stored in the memory

A calculator with a memory facility will first have a key that enables you to clear the memory (see Figure 7.1(a)). This is often labelled *MC*, standing for 'memory clear'. Always remember to press this first before you use other memory keys, to ensure the memory is empty. Strictly speaking it is not empty; it actually contains the number zero (0). Then it will have a key that you can press to display what is in the memory. This is often labelled *MR*, standing for 'memory recall'. On some calculators, the MR and MC keys are combined in an MRC key; the first press on this acts as the MR key and the second press as the MC key.

There would then be two other keys that allow you either to add what is displayed to the number stored in the memory or to subtract it. These are usually labelled *M+* and *M–*, respectively.

So, here is one way (not the only way) to calculate (47.5 × 4) – (62.5 × 3) on a basic calculator.

- First clear the memory by pressing *MC*.

- Enter '62.5 × 3 =' and get the result displayed: 187.5.

- Press *M+* to add this result to the memory.

- Enter '47.5 × 4 =' and get the result displayed: 190.
- Now subtract from this the 187.5 stored in the memory, by entering '– MR ='.

What advice would you give on using calculators in healthcare practice?

We have six pieces of advice for you.

First, do not get into the habit of relying on a calculator for even the simplest calculations. Rather get into the habit of doing basic calculations by mental and informal methods that make sense to you and which use mathematical results with which you are confident. In this way you will maintain and develop your number sense and confidence in handling numbers. (We are aware that some of the examples we use in this chapter to illustrate the way calculators work are rather easy – in practice we would expect most of them to be done by mental and informal methods.)

Second, don't be ashamed to use a calculator when the calculations are particularly tricky for you and you would not be confident that your answer is correct. What is absolutely essential is that your calculation results are accurate.

Third, an intelligent practitioner will often do some parts of a calculation mentally and some on their calculator. For example, to find '(101 – 32) ÷ 1.8' we would probably do the '101 – 32' mentally and then the division by 1.8 on the calculator.

Fourth, remember that calculators do not display 'trailing zeros' after the decimal point in results of calculations. So, a result such as 5.70 will be displayed as 5.7; 0.600 will be displayed as 0.6; 3.050 will be displayed as 3.05. For example, if you buy six batteries at £1.35 each and enter '6 × 1.35 =' to find the total cost the result displayed will be 8.1. We hope the reader would not think this means eight pounds and one penny! The cost is £8.10, but the calculator does not show the trailing zero.

EXAMPLE 7.3

A total daily dosage of 1.400 grams of a drug is to be given by slow intravenous infusion in 4 equal doses at 6-hour intervals. Each dose is calculated by entering '1.400 ÷ 4 =' on a calculator. The result displayed is 0.35. This is best written down as 0.350, so that it is clearly interpreted as 350 mg (and not 35 mg).

Fifth, as with handling any piece of technology in a healthcare context, be careful to follow standard procedures to minimize the risk of spreading infection.

Sixth, always check that a calculator result is reasonable.

How can you check that a calculator result is reasonable?

Here are five suggestions.

Checking that a calculator result is reasonable

Some ways to do this:
- repeat the calculation
- mental approximations
- set upper and lower bounds
- use inverse operations
- use professional common sense

First, it is always worth repeating a calculation you have done on a calculator and making sure that you get the same answer twice!

Second, use appropriate mental approximations. For example, when you enter '62.5 × 3 =' you would expect to see displayed a number just a bit more than 60 × 3, which you can calculate mentally as 180. So, a result of 187.5 looks reasonable.

Third, you can often set upper and lower bounds between which you know the answer must lie. For example, 62.5 × 3 must lie between 60 × 3 and 70 × 3, so you would be suspicious if the calculator result was not between 180 and 210.

EXAMPLE 7.4

Metronidazole by intravenous infusion for a child is given every 8 hours as a dose of 7.5 mg per kilogram of the child's weight; for what weight of child would the dose prescribed be 240 mg? On a calculator someone does the calculation '240 ÷ 7.5' and gets the result 42.1052632. They query this result, because they would expect the result for 240 ÷ 7.5 to lie between 30 (that's 240 ÷ 8) and 40 (that's 240 ÷ 6). The calculation is repeated and a better-looking result of 32 is displayed. They realize that they must have keyed in '240 ÷ 5.7' by mistake.

Fourth, you can apply the *inverse* operation and see if you get back to the number you started with. Multiplication and division are inverse operations (see Chapter 3). So, imagine you have calculated 62.5 × 3 and got the answer 187.5; well, if you *divide* this answer by 3 you should get back to 62.5. If you don't you have made a mistake somewhere. The person who calculated 240 ÷ 7.5 in Example 7.4 above would expect to get back to 240 if they were to *multiply* their result by 7.5. Their doubts about the answer 42.1052632 are confirmed when they find that multiplying this by 7.5 gives them a result greater than 300.

Fifth, remember to use your professional common sense! If your calculation leads to a dosage greater or less than anything you have seen before – such as too many or too few tablets, vials or bags of fluid – it is very likely that you have made a mistake in the calculation, probably just pressing the wrong keys on your calculator at some stage. Check it and check it again, or seek advice.

There's one small point to watch out for related to rounding, which we will discuss further in Chapter 8. But for now note that because calculators can display only a certain number of digits (8 or 9 is often the maximum), sometimes, particularly in a division, there can be a small *rounding error*. So, for example, in calculating the 8-hourly dose required to deliver 50 ml per day of a medicine we would enter on a calculator: 50 ÷ 3 =.

The result displayed might be either 16.6666666 or 16.6666667, depending on what your calculator does about rounding. You may then find that when you multiply your result by 3 you get a result that is either just a tiny bit less than 50 or a tiny bit more. This does not mean that you have made an error. Try this on your calculator and see what happens.

What other examples of using a calculator in healthcare contexts are there?

You would justifiably use a calculator when the calculation required is just a bit too tricky for you to feel confident that you can get the right result. Below are two examples of situations in which you might resort to a calculator and how you might check that the results are reasonable.

EXAMPLE 7.5

Drug A is prescribed at a dose of 25 mg per square metre of body surface area. A child has an estimated body surface area of 1.75 square metres. You need to calculate the correct dose of drug A for this child. The calculation required is a tricky multiplication, 25 × 1.75. So, on a calculator press this sequence of keys: '25 × 1.75 ='. The result displayed is 43.75, which represents a dosage of 43.75 mg.

This result looks reasonable because 25 × 1.75 should lie between 25 and 50, but closer to 50, because 1.75 is getting on for 2. You can also check that you have pressed the right keys on the calculator by applying the inverse operation to your result. So, if the 43.75 is still on display, divide this by 1.75 and expect to get back to the 25 you started with.

EXAMPLE 7.6

A child requires 6-hourly doses of 400 mg of phenoxymethylpenicillin. This is available in an oral suspension, which contains 125 mg of the drug in 5 millilitres. To find the volume of the drug to be administered each 6 hours we would need to calculate 400 ÷ 125 to find the number of doses of 5 ml of the suspension required, and then to multiply the result by 5. A tricky calculation! On a basic calculator we would simply press this sequence of keys: '400 ÷ 125 × 5 ='. The result displayed is 16, which means that the dose required every six hours is 16 ml of the suspension.

This result looks reasonable. A dose of 5 ml delivers 125 mg, so a dose of 15 ml (which is nearly the 16 ml in our calculator result) would deliver 375 mg (which is getting close to the 400 mg we need). Dosage examples like this involve the mathematical concept of proportionality, which is explained in detail in Chapter 12.

7.1 The drip rate for a particular intravenous infusion is 47.5 ml per hour. Use a calculator to calculate the total volume delivered over 24 hours (the calculation required is 47.5 × 24). Give the result:

(a) in millilitres   (b) in litres

How might you check that your calculator result is reasonable?

7.2 Use a calculator to divide the hourly drip rate in check-up 7.1 by 60 and hence find the drip rate in millilitres per minute.
Use an inverse operation to check your result.

7.3 The 8-hourly dose of metronidazole by intravenous infusion for a child of weight 29 kg is 29 × 7.5 mg. Use a calculator to work this out. Give the dose:

(a) in milligrams   (b) in grams

How might you check mentally that your result is reasonable?

7.4 How might you use the memory facility on a basic calculator to help you do the calculation 12 × 4 + 16 × 2, used earlier in this chapter in Example 7.1 for working out the total number of tablets required by the patient over a four-week period?

7.5 Prednisolone is a drug used in the treatment of many inflammatory diseases and it is often used with a reducing regime over a period of weeks. The tablets dispensed are 5 mg. A typical regime for six weeks of treatment would be

6 tablets per day for 7 days; then

5 tablets per day for the next 7 days; then

4 tablets per day for the next 7 days; then

3 tablets per day for the next 7 days; then

2 tablets per day for the next 7 days; then

1 tablet per day for the final 7 days.

We need to calculate how many tablets are required in total for the whole 6 weeks treatment. The calculation required here could be expressed like this, with the multiplications assumed to take precedence over the additions:

$$7 \times 6 + 7 \times 5 + 7 \times 4 + 7 \times 3 + 7 \times 2 + 7.$$

For the purpose of this exercise, ignore the fact that you could do this calculation mentally!

(a) What key sequence would do this on a scientific calculator?

(b) How could you do this on a basic calculator, making use of the memory facility?

ROUNDING

8

OBJECTIVES

In a practical healthcare context the practitioner should be able to:

- read measurements of time, liquid volume, weight and temperature to an appropriate degree of accuracy
- recognize that all measurements are approximate, being limited by the level of precision possible for the measuring device used
- round numbers and measurements up or down or to the nearest whole number, ten, or hundred, and so on
- round numbers and measurements to a given number of decimal places
- round numbers and measurements to a given number of significant digits
- be aware of rounding errors in calculations
- use rounding to check the reasonableness of the result of a calculation

In this chapter we use a number of practical illustrations, such as dosage calculations and infusion rates, which are explained in detail in later chapters. In this chapter we intend the reader just to focus on the ways on which results of calculations are rounded.

SPOT THE ERRORS

Identify any obvious errors in rounding numbers or measurements in the following ten statements.

  1 The syringe depicted in Figure 8.1 contains exactly 6.5 ml of fluid.

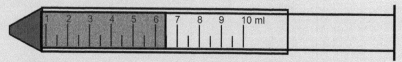

Figure 8.1 How much fluid is contained in this syringe?

  2 The syringe depicted in Figure 8.1 contains 6.5 ml of fluid to the nearest half millimetre.
  3 The arrow in Figure 8.2 shows the height of a woman on a measuring scale; her height is 157 cm to the nearest centimetre.

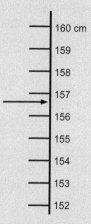

Figure 8.2 Indication of the height of a woman on a measuring scale

  4 A patient is prescribed a blood transfusion of 500 ml of blood. This is equivalent to receiving 7500 drops of blood. These are to be delivered over 240 minutes. To find the number of drops to be infused per minute, this calculation is entered on a calculator: 7500 ÷ 240 = 31.25. This result is rounded to 31 drops per minute.
  5 An infusion of dextrose 5% has 772 ml remaining. This is now to be infused over the next 6 hours.

Using a calculator, 772 ÷ 6 = 128.666667, so the infusion rate to be set is 129 ml per hour, rounded to the nearest millilitre.

6   In one year the Norfolk and Norwich University Hospitals NHS Foundation Trust treated 729 488 patients. To the nearest ten thousand this number is 730 000 patients.

7   Rounded to three significant digits the number of patients given in Statement 6 above is 729 000 patients.

8   A 50-ml serving of skimmed milk contains 0.0645 grams of calcium; rounded to two decimal places this is 0.06 grams.

9   Rounded to three significant digits the weight of calcium given in Statement 8 is 0.065 grams.

10 A patient is prescribed 3000 micrograms of morphine over 24 hours. Dividing 3000 by 24, a nurse calculates that the patient requires 12.5 micrograms per hour.

Are the errors you have spotted potentially serious in medical health practice?

(errors identified over the page)

Is it possible to make an exact measurement?

In practice every measurement we make is only as accurate as is possible within the limitations of the measuring device we are using, whether it be, for example, a tape measure, a set of weighing scales, a thermometer, or a syringe. You may think when you buy 500 grams of butter, for example, that you have every right to expect to get 'exactly' 500 grams of butter. But if you look closely at the pack you will find a symbol looking like a large lower case letter *e*. This symbol appears on most packages of items sold by weight or volume and is a European Union indication that the quantity can be guaranteed to lie only within certain mandatory limits. It is a reminder that no measurement can be exact. It can only ever be made 'to the nearest something'. Having said that, we will always aim to make our measurements as accurate as is possible within the constraints of our equipment and to record them to whatever level of precision is appropriate.

The limitations of the measuring device

All measurements of such variables as weight, volume and temperature can be only as accurate as possible within the limitations of the piece of equipment being used to make the measurement.

What is measuring 'to the nearest something'?

In everyday life we often round numbers to the nearest something. For example, someone who has an annual salary of £30 864 might say that their salary is 'about £31 000'.

ERRORS IDENTIFIED

The obvious errors are Statements 1, 9 and 10.

Statement 1

What is wrong with this statement is the word 'exactly'. As we explain below, all measurements are in fact approximate; they are always made 'to the nearest something' (as in Statement 2) or to a specified level of accuracy. Statement 1 is not a serious error in medical health practice, although overhearing it may initiate an acute medical condition in a pedantic mathematician (like one of the authors).

Statement 9

The weight of 0.0645 grams is already rounded to three significant digits. The idea of significant digits is explained below. In this case the first non-zero digit reading from the left is the '6'. This is the first significant digit; the 4 and the 5 are the second and third significant digits, respectively. This kind of error would be serious in a medical research context where small variations in recorded data might be important and the third significant digits in measurements are required to register these.

Statement 10

The calculation is clearly incorrect. To see this, round the 24 to 20, just to get a very approximate result using a calculation that is easy to do mentally: 3000 ÷ 20 is equivalent to 300 ÷ 2, which is 150. So we would be expecting an answer in the region of 150 micrograms. This suggests that the result 12.5 micrograms is wrong and the calculation should be done again. The correct result is 125 micrograms. The error in Statement 10 is potentially a serious error in a dosage calculation.

(now continue reading from page 85)

They have rounded the number to the nearest thousand. The salary of £30 864 lies between £30 000 and £31 000, but it is nearer to 31 000 than it is to 30 000. Similarly, a hospital manager might respond to a question about how many consultants are employed by the hospital by saying 'about 350', when the actual number is 339: in this case the manager may have thought it sufficient to round the number to the nearest fifty.

We do the same kind of thing with measurements. A man may say that he is 182 cm tall, when to be precise he should say he is '182 cm tall to the nearest centimetre'. To make this statement there are two steps involved, as illustrated in Figure 8.3:

Two steps in rounding

(a) identify which two points on the scale the number (or measurement) lies between;
(b) decide which of these is nearer to the number being rounded.

(a) identify which of the two centimetre marks on the scale the man's height lies between;
(b) decide which of these is nearer to his height.

In this case the man's height (a) lies between 181 cm and 182 cm, and (b) is nearer to 182 cm than it is to 181 cm.

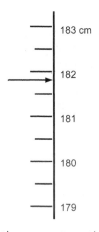

Figure 8.3   Measuring to the nearest centimetre

Rounding to the nearest something

Figure 8.3 shows us that any height that falls between 181.5 cm and 182.5 cm would be recorded as 182 cm to the nearest centimetre, because any height in this range would be nearer to 182 cm than either of 181 cm or 183 cm. See also Figure 8.2 and the (correct) Statement 3 in *Spot the errors* at the start of this chapter, where the woman's height is between 156 cm and 157 cm, but nearer to 157 cm. The healthcare practitioner will encounter many situations like these in which numbers and measurements that arise in their practice have to be rounded in some way.

Measurements might be rounded, for example, to

• the nearest whole unit,
• the nearest half a unit (0.5),
• the nearest tenth of a unit (0.1), and so on.

There is a range of values that round to the same value.

EXAMPLE 8.1

A 12-hour infusion is set up to deliver 1000 ml of a solution of sodium chloride 0.9% (this use of percentages to describe the concentration of a solution is explained in Chapter 13). A nurse calculates that the infusion would require 83.333333 ml to be delivered each hour. (The calculation done on a calculator is: 1000 ÷ 12 = 83.333333.) The calculator result (83.333333) is already truncated to the number of digits that it can display. But, in practice, it is not possible to set an infusion rate to anything like this level of accuracy – nor would it be necessary or appropriate. It is quite sufficient in this example to round this result to the nearest millilitre and to use this, without any risk to the patient's well-being. The result rounded to the nearest millilitre is 83 ml to be delivered each hour.

(We discuss the calculation of infusion rates more fully in Chapter 12.)

The phrase 'to the nearest something' suggests that we are dealing with a spatial idea. It is helpful therefore to have in mind a picture of an appropriate section of a number line, as shown in Figure 8.4. This shows the range of values – between 82.5 ml and 83.5 ml – that are nearer to 83 ml than to any other whole number of millilitres. So, any value in this range is rounded to 83 ml when rounding to the nearest millilitre. The volume 83.333333 ml would lie somewhere between 83 and 83.5 ml, so this is *rounded down* to 83 ml.

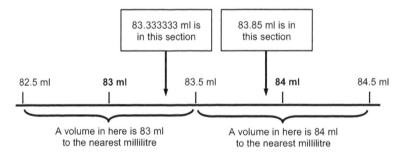

Figure 8.4   Rounding to the nearest millilitre

If, however, a calculation had given an infusion rate of, say, 83.65 ml per hour, then Figure 8.4 shows that this volume is in the range of values that are nearer to 84 ml than to any other whole number of millilitres. So this value would be *rounded up* to 84 ml to the nearest millilitre.

EXAMPLE 8.2

A man attending a diabetic clinic is weighed every six months. The scales being used give the measurement to the nearest half a kilogram (that is, 0.5 kg). On one appointment the digital scales give his weight as 77.5 kg. Six months earlier his weight had been recorded as 78.5 kg. The nurse tells him he has lost 1 kilogram in weight. Is the nurse correct?

No! We will explain. This measuring device is not designed to give a measurement of any greater accuracy than the nearest half a kilogram. So, for example, from 75 kg to 80 kg, the scales can give only these readings: 75.0, 75.5, 76.0, 76.5, 77.0, 77.5, 78.0, 78.5, 79.0, 79.5, 80.0. This is sufficiently accurate; in practice, a change of half a kilogram or less in an adult's recorded body weight is not likely to be of much significance, given variations in things such as fluid retention, the time of day and the weight of socks.

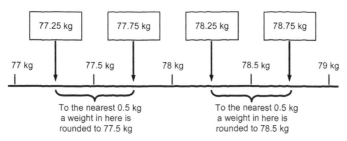

Figure 8.5 Number line showing weights from 77 kg to 79 kg

Figure 8.5 is a section of a number line, showing weights from 77 kg to 79 kg; the scale goes up by half a kilogram (0.5 kg) from one mark to the next. We can see from this diagram that a weight recorded as 77.5 kg to the nearest half a kilogram could be anywhere between 77.25 kg and 77.75 kg. A weight recorded as 78.5 kg could be anywhere between 78.25 kg and 78.75 kg. Figure 8.5 shows that the two weights recorded as 77.5 kg and 78.5 kg to the nearest half a kilogram could differ by any amount between 0.5 kg (78.25 kg – 77.75 kg) and 1.5 kg (78.75 kg – 77.25 kg)! The nurse in Example 8.2 has made the calculation of the change in weight as though the measurements were exact.

EXAMPLE 8.3

A digital thermometer is used every half an hour to measure a patient's temperature. The thermometer being used gives the temperature to the nearest tenth of a degree (that is, 0.1 degrees). Over three hours the readings are: 38.5°, 38.4°, 38.0°, 37.9°, 37.6° and 37.1°. All the readings from this thermometer will have a single digit after the decimal point like these readings. A temperature around 38.44°, for example, would be rounded down automatically by the thermometer to give a reading of 38.4° to the nearest tenth of a degree (see Figure 8.6). This is because 38.44 lies between 38.4 (38.40) and 38.5 (38.50), but it is nearer to 38.4. A temperature around 38.36° would be rounded up to give the same reading of 38.4° to the nearest tenth of a degree. This is because 38.36 lies between 38.3 (38.30) and 38.4 (38.40), but is nearer to 38.4.

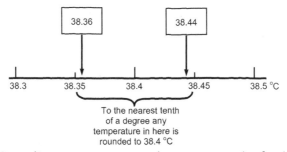

Figure 8.6 Rounding temperatures to the nearest tenth of a degree

Some readers will no doubt be thinking, but what do you do when the number you are rounding is exactly halfway between two possible values? For example, how would you round 67.5 ml to the nearest ml? That's as near to 67 ml as it is to 68 ml. There is no one answer to this question that applies in every situation. In practice, sometimes you will round it down to 67 ml, sometimes round it up to 68 ml; see the next section. If it is practical, just leave it as 67.5 ml.

Is rounding always done to the nearest something?

It is interesting to note that there are situations where you always round up and never round down. For example, you will always round up in any question that asks how many or how much do you need to achieve a target. Here's a simple example of what we mean.

EXAMPLE 8.4

A pharmacy supplies boxes of paracetamol containing 16 tablets. How many boxes would be needed to meet a requirement for 84 tablets? If 84 is divided by 16 the result (5.25) indicates that 5.25 boxes are required. This number will be rounded up to 6 boxes. The context here makes clear that we have to round this result up to 6 boxes, even though the result is nearer to 5 than to 6. With 5 boxes we would fall short of the required 84 tablets.

Similarly, there are situations where you always round down and never round up. If you are aiming to catch the 10.47 train, you would be advised to round this time down (to, say, 10.40) rather than up (to, say, 10.50) in planning to get to the station! You'll be pleased to know, for example, that when the UK tax authorities are calculating your income tax they always round *down* your income to the nearest pound below. Here's another simple example to illustrate this point.

EXAMPLE 8.5

How many doses of 30 ml are available in 500 ml of a solution? If 500 is divided by 30 the result indicates that 16.666667 doses are available. This number has to be rounded down to 16 doses. The context here makes it obvious that we have to round this result down to 16 doses, even though 16.666667 is nearer to 17 than to 16. There is not sufficient for 17 doses.

The point we are making is that the context of the calculation is the first consideration when deciding whether to round up or round down. For example, for an adult patient small additional volumes of fluid arising from rounding up are not likely to be as significant clinically as they would be in a neonate or small child – when it might be safer to adopt a policy of rounding down.

In some cases it is more appropriate to round numbers and measurements to a particular number of decimal places. You may also encounter the idea of rounding to a number of significant digits. These ideas are explained below.

How do you round to a number of decimal places?

In some contexts the limitations of the measuring equipment or simply a recognition of what level of accuracy is appropriate require that a quantity is rounded to a certain number of decimal places. We described the rounding in Example 8.3 above as rounding to the nearest tenth of a degree. We could also describe this as 'rounding to one decimal place'. This is because each temperature is given with one digit after the decimal place.

Rounding up or down?

The context that gives rise to a calculation is the first consideration in deciding whether it is more appropriate to round a result up or to round it down.

Rounding to a number of decimal places

Rounding the number 8.13579 ...

- to one decimal place gives 8.1;
- to two decimal places gives 8.14;
- to three decimal places gives 8.136;
- and to four decimal places gives 8.1358.

EXAMPLE 8.6

The infusion rate for delivering 1 litre of a solution of dextrose 5% (see Chapter 13 for the meaning of this 5%) to an adult patient over 6 hours is calculated to be $1000 \div 6 = 166.66667$ ml per hour. Dividing this by 60 on a calculator, a nurse finds that this is equivalent to 2.7777778 ml per minute. This is rounded to one decimal place, giving a drip rate of 2.8 ml per minute. (We give further explanations of the calculations required in examples like this in Chapter 12.) The equipment being used cannot be set to any greater accuracy than to one tenth of a millilitre– nor would any greater accuracy be necessary in this practical context – in other words only one digit can be used after the decimal place. Rounding the result to one decimal place in this example involves these two steps:

(a) recognizing that 2.7777778 lies between 2.7 and 2.8;
(b) deciding that it is nearer to 2.8 than it is to 2.7.

In step (b) it is helpful to note that halfway between 2.7 and 2.8 is 2.75, and a number starting 2.77… is greater than this.

EXAMPLE 8.7

A woman is 1.63 metres in height and has a weight of 64.5 kilograms. Her 'body-mass index' (see Chapter 14) is calculated as $64.5 \div (1.63 \times 1.63)$. A calculator gives this result as 24.276412. It would be inappropriate to give a body-mass index to six decimal places, since this implies a level of accuracy far beyond what is possible with the raw data involved. So, in practice this result would probably be rounded to one decimal place and recorded as 24.3.

For the purposes of illustration we will also round the result 24.276412 to two decimal places. This gives us 24.28. This rounding involves these two steps:

(a) recognizing that 24.276412 lies between 24.27 and 24.28;
(b) deciding that it is nearer to 24.28 than it is to 24.27.

In step (b) it is helpful to note that halfway between 24.27 and 24.28 is 24.275, and a number starting 24.276… is greater than this.

EXAMPLE 8.8

A calculation of a drip rate for an infusion gives the result 2.975 ml per minute. What is this rounded to one decimal place? This result (2.975) lies between 2.9 and 3.0, but it is greater than 2.95 and therefore is closer to 3.0. Rounded to one decimal place the drip rate is therefore 3.0 ml. Note that it is good mathematical practice to record this as 3.0 ml rather than 3 ml. Retaining the zero after the decimal point is an indication that the volume has been rounded to one decimal place. (Recording it as 3 ml would indicate that the volume had been rounded to the nearest millilitre.)

What is meant by rounding to a number of significant digits?

Significant digits 12.3456

In the number 12.3456, the first significant digit is the digit 1, the second is the 2, the third is the 3, and so on.

Rounded to three significant digits the number is 12.3.

What is an appropriate level of rounding? To the nearest whole number? To one decimal place? To two decimal places? One of the considerations in answering this question is how large or small are the numbers involved. For example, consider these results of three calculations of dosages of morphine: 0.125mg, 0.140mg and 0.13333333 mg (or, expressed in micrograms, 125 micrograms, 140 micrograms and 133.33333 micrograms). If these were rounded to the nearest whole number of milligrams they would all be zero! Even if the measurements in milligrams were rounded to one decimal place they would all be the same: 0.1 mg. It is often sensible to round numbers and measurements in a way that retains *three significant digits*. This ensures that we do not throw away too much of the number when we round it. In this illustration, the three dosages rounded to three significant digits in milligrams are 0.125 mg, 0.140 mg and 0.133 mg. Expressing these dosages in micrograms to three significant digits we get precisely the same three digits in each case: 125 micrograms, 140 micrograms and 133 micrograms.

Significant digits
0.00123456

In the number 0.00123456, the first significant digit is again the digit 1, the second is the 2, the third is the 3, and so on.

Rounded to three significant digits the number is 0.00123.

The first significant digit in a number is the first non-zero digit as you read the number from left to right. The subsequent digits (including any zeros) are the second, third, fourth (and so on) significant digits. The idea is that as you read a number from left to right the digits you encounter get less and less significant, so we just retain the first three of them (not counting any leading zeros).

So, for example, in the volume 23.875 ml the 2 at the beginning (which stands for twenty millilitres) is much more significant than the 5 at the end (which stands for five thousandths of a millilitre). To round 23.875 ml to three significant digits, we discard everything after the 8. But before we do this, we decide whether the 8 gets rounded up to 9 or not. Since the number is closer to 23.9 than to 23.8, rounded to three significant digits the volume of 23.875 ml becomes 23.9 ml.

Notice that if this same volume had been given in litres it would have been 0.023875 litres. The first significant digit (the first non-zero digit from the left) is again the 2. So, rounded to three significant digits this volume is 0.0239 litres – which is the same volume as 23.9 ml!

In many practical contexts a measurement with three significant digits is as accurate as you need to be.

EXAMPLE 8.9

Some examples of rounding results of calculations to three significant digits:

- A dosage calculated as 426.4 mg is rounded to 426 mg
- A monthly salary of £2567.85 is rounded to £2570
- A volume of 0.0756667 litres is rounded to 0.0757 litres
- The same volume expressed in millilitres (75.6667 ml) is rounded to 75.7 ml
- A body-mass index calculated as 29.0285 is rounded to 29.0

If a lower level of precision is acceptable then numbers can be rounded to two significant digits: the principle is the same. Similarly, four (or more) significant digits could be used for greater precision. For example, the body-mass index of 29.0285 rounded to two significant digits is 29 and rounded to four significant digits is 29.03.

What about other examples of rounding in healthcare contexts?

The calculations required in Examples 8.10 – 8.12 below are explained in more detail in Chapter 12. Here we are focusing on the process of rounding.

EXAMPLE 8.10

An adult weighing 63.5 kg is prescribed a dose of acetylcysteine and this is calculated as a volume of 15.875 ml. This is added to 500 ml of 5% dextrose, giving a total volume 515.875 ml. This volume of liquid is to be infused over a period of 4 hours. The infusion rate required per hour to deliver 515.875 ml over 4 hours is calculated as 515.875 ÷ 4 = 128.96875 ml per hour. An infusion pump cannot be set to this level of precision. The volume of 128.96875 ml must therefore be rounded to the nearest millilitre. The number 128.96875 lies between 128 and 129, but is closer to 129. The infusion rate to be set is 129 ml per hour.

EXAMPLE 8.11

A child requires 250 mg of paracetamol as a single dose. Paracetamol is available as a suspension containing 24 mg in 1 ml. The calculation required to find the volume to be given to the child is 250 ÷ 24, which on a calculator gives the result 10.416667. This must be rounded to one decimal place. A volume of 10.416667 ml lies between 10.4 ml and 10.5 ml, but it is closer to 10.4 ml. So, rounding to one decimal place, we find the volume required to be 10.4 ml.

EXAMPLE 8.12

A volume of 500 ml of a solution of sodium chloride 0.9% is to be infused over 6 hours. Calculate the volume to be infused per hour (a) in litres, (b) in millilitres, in each case giving the result to three significant digits. Compare the results.

(a) Taking the volume as 0.5 litres, we divide 0.5 by 6, giving a result of 0.0833333 litres per hour To three significant digits this is 0.0833 litres per hour.

(b) Taking the volume as 500 ml, we divide 500 by 6, giving a result of 83.33333 ml per hour. To three significant digits this is 83.3 ml per hour.

The two results are the same! 0.0833 litres= 83.3 ml.

What are rounding errors?

Clearly, whenever we round a result or a measurement in some way we are introducing a small error in the value. We saw in Chapter 7 an example of a rounding error in using a calculator, resulting from the fact that a calculator may have to round an answer in some way because it can only display 8 or 9 digits.

Rounding errors

Rounding introduces a small error in results. Be aware that sometimes this might be significant. Avoid using rounded data in subsequent calculations, because small errors can be magnified in the process to large ones.

We will look briefly at the effects of the rounding errors produced by some of the examples in this chapter.

In Example 8.1, the result, 83.33333 ml per hour, was rounded to 83 ml per hour. By rounding we have introduced a very small error, just 0.333333 ml. But what is the effect of that on the time it takes to infuse the whole litre of fluid? We can calculate how long it will take to infuse 1000 ml at the rate of 83 ml per hour, by dividing 1000 by 83. The result is 12.05 hours (rounded to two decimal places), or about 12 hours and 3 minutes. The plan was to deliver the 1000 ml in 12 hours. The extra 3 minutes is the effect of rounding. This calculation shows how a very small error introduced in the rounding process can potentially be quite noticeable when multiplied a large number of times. Having said that, however, we can be reassured in this case that the extra 3 minutes are not significant in terms of the well-being of the patient.

In Example 8.6, the calculated drip rate of 2.7777778 ml per minute was rounded to 2.8 ml per minute. Because we have rounded up here it means that the litre of fluid will be delivered slightly quicker than required. But how much quicker? If we divide the 1000 ml by 2.8 ml ($1000 \div 2.8 = 357.142857$) we find that the litre of fluid is infused in just over 357 minutes, which is about 3 minutes quicker than planned. Again, a very small error introduced in rounding has produced a noticeable effect in the long run. So it is worth considering the effect of rounding errors, even if it is just to reassure ourselves – as in this case – that it is not significant in terms of the patient's well-being.

Example 8.2 in this chapter is another illustration of the effect of rounding errors. This illustrates the key point that we need to be aware of: the problem of using rounded values in subsequent calculations. In this example, you cannot say that two weights given to the nearest half a kilogram as 77.5 kg and 78.5 kg respectively differ by 1 kilogram! Consider these two examples: (a) the first weight might actually be 77.26 kg and the second one might be 78.74 kg, in which case they would differ by 1.48 kg; (b) the first weight might actually be 77.74 kg and the second one might be 78.26 kg, in which case they would differ by 0.52 kg!

Example 8.13 below is an illustration of the way in which rounding errors can accumulate. This is not given as an example to follow, but as a warning!

EXAMPLE 8.13

(Illustrating the danger of accumulating rounding errors)

Drug A is prescribed for a child on the basis of the patient's body surface area measured in square metres. Body surface area is calculated by a formula involving

(Continued)

(Continued)

the child's height in metres and weight in kilograms (see Chapter 14).

The dosage of Drug A is 50 mg for each square metre of body surface area.

The child's height and weight are measured as accurately as possible as 101.6 cm and 14.52 kg. Assume that each of these is rounded to the nearest unit, giving 102 cm and 15 kg respectively. The formula (explained in Chapter 14) for calculating body surface area gives a result of 0.6519. Assume that this is then rounded to one decimal place as 0.7. The dosage is then calculated as $50 \times 0.7 = 35$ mg.

If, however, the unrounded numbers are used throughout this calculation the final result for the dosage turns out to be only 32 mg. That is a 3-mg lower dosage of Drug A.

The message here is this: as far as possible, when a precise calculation is required avoid introducing rounding errors in the data being used for subsequent calculations. Wait until you have the final answer before you do any rounding.

How do you use rounding to check the reasonableness of the results of calculations?

EXAMPLE 8.14

(a) In Example 8.11 it was found that 10.4 ml of a suspension containing 24 mg of paracetamol in 1 ml was required to deliver 250 mg of paracetamol. Is this a reasonable result? To check this, we could mentally round 10.4 ml to 10 ml, and think: 'If 1 ml contains 24 g, then 10 ml will contain 240 mg, which is just a bit short of the 250 mg required.' So the result 10.4 ml looks reasonable.

(b) A practitioner calculates that the infusion of 1000 ml of fluid over 6 hours requires a drip rate of 16.7 ml per hour. Does this result look reasonable? Mentally, the practitioner rounds 16.7 ml to the nearest 10 ml, to get 20 ml. A drip rate of 20 ml per hour is only 120 ml in 6 hours! That's a long way short of the required 1000 ml. The calculation is repeated and the (correct) result is found to be 166.66667 ml per hour, which is rounded to 167 ml per hour.

8.1 Figure 8.7 shows three syringes (a), (b) and (c). In each case write down the volume of fluid drawn by the syringe to the nearest half a millilitre (0.5 of a millilitre).

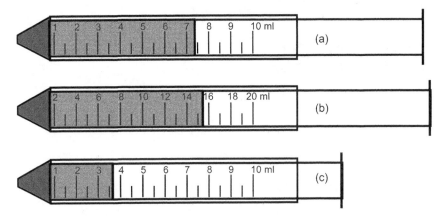

Figure 8.7   Read the volumes drawn to the nearest half a millilitre (check-up question 8.1)

8.2 The result of a dosage calculation is 27.096667 mg. What is this dose:

(a) rounded to the nearest milligram?
(b) rounded to one decimal place?
(c) rounded to two decimal places?
(d) rounded to three significant digits?

8.3 The result of a dosage calculation is 0.08764 g. What is this dose:

(a) rounded to one decimal place?
(b) rounded to two decimal places?
(c) rounded to three decimal places?
(d) rounded to three significant digits?

8.4 If the dosage required in Example 8.11 (earlier in the chapter) were 375 mg of paracetamol, to find the volume of suspension in millilitres the calculation required would be 375 ÷ 24. Do this calculation on a calculator and round the answer to the nearest millilitre.

8.5 The next stage of treatment for the patient in Example 8.10 (earlier in the chapter) requires a total volume of 1031.75 ml to be infused over a period of 16 hours. The calculation required to find the infusion rate in millilitres per hour is 1031.75 ÷ 16. Do this on a calculator. Round the result and give the infusion rate to the nearest millilitre per hour.

8.6 On a calculator, divide 1031.75 by your answer to check-up question 8.5. This will give you the time in hours that it will take to deliver the total volume prescribed. Why is this more than 16 hours?

CALCULATIONS WITH DECIMAL NUMBERS 9

OBJECTIVES

In a practical healthcare context the practitioner should be able to:

- mentally add and subtract decimal numbers with just one or two non-zero digits
- perform accurately additions and subtractions involving decimal numbers
- perform accurately straightforward multiplications involving decimal numbers
- perform accurately straightforward divisions involving decimal numbers
- check the reasonableness of the answer to a multiplication or division calculation involving decimal numbers and recognize when it is clearly incorrect

Note that in this chapter and elsewhere in this book we use the term *decimal number* to refer to any number that has one or more non-zero digits after the decimal point. The examples used in this chapter are indicative of the kinds of calculations with decimal numbers that a numerate practitioner should find straightforward, without recourse to a calculator. We use a number of examples from healthcare contexts that are explained in later chapters; but here the focus is on the actual calculations, rather than on knowing what calculations to do.

SPOT THE ERRORS

Identify any obvious errors in the following ten statements.

1 A patient who has drunk a 0.25 ml glass of water followed by a further 0.15 ml of water has drunk 0.4 ml of water altogether in the two drinks.

2 If a 3-litre container of an irrigation fluid has 1.35 litres remaining in it, then a volume of 1.65 litres has been already taken out of it.

3 When a volume of 0.024 litres of iron dextran is added to 0.75 litres of sodium chloride solution the total volume is 0.99 litres.

4 A patient who is prescribed 1.6 mg of morphine per hour by infusion and who has so far received 1.38 mg of the hourly dose requires a further 0.32 mg.

5 If an ampoule contains 0.04 g of Drug A, then 6 ampoules will contain a total of 0.24 g of Drug A.

6 Drug B is prescribed at a dose of 25 milligrams for each square metre of body surface area. A patient with an estimated body surface area of 1.8 square metres will therefore require 25 × 1.8 mg of Drug B, which equals 25.200 mg.

7 The answer to 85 ÷ 0.9125 is greater than 85.

8 If Drug C is to be given by slow intravenous infusion at a total dose of 0.225 g per kilogram of body weight, the total dose for a neonate weighing 4 kg is 4 × 0.225 g, which equals 0.9 g.

9 If a total of 0.9 g of Drug D is to be given in three equal doses then each dose must be 0.3 g.

10 If 1.8 g of Drug E is prescribed and each tablet contains 0.3 g of Drug E, then the number of tablets required is 60.

Are the errors you have spotted potentially serious in medical health practice?

(errors identified over the page)

ERRORS IDENTIFIED

The obvious errors are Statements 3, 4, 6 and 10. All the errors here are potentially serious: the accurate prescription and administration of drugs is fundamental to good healthcare practice.

Statement 3

The sum of 0.024 and 0.75 is not 0.99 litres. Below we explain how to avoid this kind of error by ensuring that each number has the same number of digits after the decimal point. So, this addition becomes 0.024 + 0.750, which equals 0.774. So the total volume is 0.774 litres.

Statement 4

The calculation required here is 1.6 – 1.38. This may helpfully be written as 1.60 – 1.38, with the same numbers of digits after the decimal point in each number. We discuss below various ways in which this kind of subtraction might be done to achieve the correct answer, 0.22.

Statement 6

The reader should spot that the result here (25.200 mg) is wrong because it just looks too small. Rounding the 1.8 to 2, we would expect the result for 25 × 1.8 mg to be closer to 25 × 2 mg, which is 50 mg. We explain ways of doing multiplications involving decimals (like 25 × 1.8) later in this chapter.

Statement 10

If 1.8 g of Drug E is prescribed and each tablet contains 0.3 g of Drug E, then to find the number of tablets required the calculation is 1.8 ÷ 0.3. We explain below that this is equivalent to 18 ÷ 3, which is 6. Just 6 tablets are needed, not 60! This is a very serious error, but it is also possibly the most common error in drug calculations: getting the answer wrong by a factor of 10.

What kind of additions and subtractions with decimal numbers should a practitioner be able to do mentally?

Any addition and subtraction that you would expect to do mentally with whole numbers you should expect to be able to do with the same digits in decimal numbers. The principles of place value (see Chapters 1–3) apply in just the same way. You just have to keep a close eye on where the decimal point is.

For example, we expect that you can add two single digit numbers, such as: 8 + 5 = 13. So, you can do these additions with decimal numbers, because they are the same calculation but with the decimal point just shifted to a different position in the two numbers being added and consequently in the result:

(a) 0.8 + 0.5 = 1.3

(b) 0.08 + 0.05 = 0.13

(c) 0.008 + 0.005 = 0.013, and so on.

In (a) we are adding 8 tenths to 5 tenths and getting 13 tenths – that is 1 whole unit and 3 tenths, which is 1.3. In (b) we are adding 8 hundredths to 5 hundredths and getting 13 hundredths; and in (c) we are adding 8 thousandths to 5 thousandths and getting 13 thousandths.

Similarly with subtraction: you know, for example, that 25 – 12 = 13.

Keeping an eye on the position of the decimal points, you should then immediately be able to do these subtractions with decimal numbers:

(d) 2.5 – 1.2 = 1.3

(e) 0.25 – 0.12 = 0.13

(f) 0.025 – 0.012 = 0.013, and so on.

EXAMPLE 9.1

A patient is currently prescribed a dose of 0.45 mg of Drug F. Following a medical review this is decreased by 0.15 mg. To what dose is it decreased? Answer: it has been decreased to 0.30 mg.

The calculation required is 0.45 – 0.15. This is the same as calculating 45 – 15, but with the decimal point shifted two places to the left. Since we know 45 – 15 = 30, we can deduce that 0.45 – 0.15 = 0.30 g (which may also be written as 0.3 g, of course, or 300 mg).

Strategy 1

When adding and subtracting with decimal numbers it is much easier if the numbers have the same number of digits after the decimal point. If necessary, put in extra zeros at the end of one of the numbers to achieve this.

The examples above have the same number of digits after the decimal point, which makes it fairly easy to make the connection with the corresponding calculations with whole numbers. But what about calculating, say, 0.7 + 0.45? Here comes an important strategy: when adding or subtracting two numbers involving decimals, put in whatever additional zeros are needed to give the same number of digits after the decimal points! So, we rewrite 0.7 + 0.45 as 0.70 + 0.45. We can now relate this mentally to 70 + 45 = 115: so, 0.7 + 0.45 = 0.70 + 0.45 = 1.15.

EXAMPLE 9.2

A patient is on a dose of 0.5 mg of Drug F. This is decreased by 0.15 mg. To what is it decreased? Answer: it has been decreased to 0.35 mg.

The calculation required is 0.5 – 0.15. Write this as 0.50 – 0.15 and it becomes a simple calculation! This is the same as calculating 50 – 15, but with the decimal point shifted two places to the left. Since we know 50 – 15 = 35, we can deduce that 0.50 – 0.15 = 0.35.

EXAMPLE 9.3

A nurse draws 0.015 litres of blood from a patient in one syringe and 0.02 litres in another. What is the total volume drawn? Answer: a total of 0.035 litres has been drawn.

The calculation required is 0.015 + 0.02. Write this as 0.015 + 0.020, so that there are now three digits after the decimal point in each number. This is now the same as calculating 15 + 20, but with the decimal point shifted three places to the left. Since we know 15 + 20 = 35, then we deduce that 0.015 + 0.020 = 0.035.

Strategy 2

A calculation with decimal numbers can often be changed to one with whole numbers simply by rewriting the data in smaller units (such as millilitres instead of litres, micrograms instead of milligrams)

The reader may well have been wondering why we did not give the measurements in Example 9.3 in millilitres rather than in litres, because it would have been so much easier! If so, give yourself a pat on the back. This is another important strategy: you can often change a calculation involving decimal numbers into one using whole numbers, by changing the units of measurement.

So, in Example 9.3, if we write the volumes in millilitres the calculation becomes 15 ml + 20 ml = 35 ml (which can then be converted back to litres, if required, as 0.035 litres).

In Example 9.1, if we write the weights in micrograms the calculation becomes 450 – 150 = 300 micrograms (which can then be converted back to milligrams as 0.300 mg, or 0.3 mg).

In Example 9.2, writing the weights in micrograms again makes the calculation very simple: 500 micrograms – 150 micrograms = 350 micrograms (which is 0.350 mg, or 0.35 mg).

What do I need to know about addition and subtraction calculations involving decimal numbers with several digits?

We hope that you are getting the idea that the principles and procedures for addition and subtraction with decimal numbers are essentially no different from those for whole numbers. For example, calculating 3.65 + 2.75 is no different from calculating 365 + 275, apart from recognizing the position of the decimal point.

Compare the two calculations done by an informal method:

Column addition with decimals

This is just the same as with whole numbers, but with one additional thing to remember: make sure the decimal points are lined up!

(a) 365 + 275= (300 + 200) + (60 + 70) + (5 + 5)= 500 + 130 + 10 = 640

(b) 3.65 + 2.75 = (3 + 2) + (0.6 + 0.7) + (0.05 + 0.05) = 5 + 1.3 + 0.1 = 6.40

The reader should see that the calculations involved here are exactly the same, except that in (b) the decimal point is positioned two places to the left in each of the numbers involved. So, for example, where in (a) we are adding 60 and 70, in (b) we are adding 0.6 and 0.7.

Or, compare the calculations done by a formal written method (see Chapter 2):

```
  3 6 5              3.6 5
+ 2 7 5            + 2.7 5
 _____             _____
  6 4 0              6.4 0
```

You can go wrong with this only if you are careless about lining up the points and the digits either side of them!

EXAMPLE 9.4

In Spot the errors Statement 4 the calculation required is 1.6 – 1.38. Using strategy 2 above, this becomes 1.60 – 1.38.

Doing the calculation by an informal method: this is just like having £1.60 and spending £1.38. Adding on from £1.38 to get to £1.60, you get 22p change (£0.22). So 1.60 – 1.38 = 0.22. So, in Statement 4, a further 0.22 mg is required.

Figure 9.1 shows the parallel between 160 – 138 and 1.60 – 1.38, each done by the same process of 'adding on'.

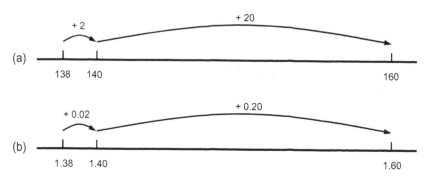

Figure 9.1   Comparing (a) 160 – 138 and (b) 1.60 – 1.38

EXAMPLE 9.5

A patient's fluid balance chart is completed up to midday to determine the total fluid intake over the past 12 hours. So far today the patient has received 1.5 litres of fluid by intravenous infusion and a total oral intake of 145 ml. What is the patient's total fluid intake to midday today, in litres?

Reminder about units

Make sure that quantities being added or subtracted are in the same units. For example: all litres or all millilitres; all grams or all milligrams or all micrograms.

Before we do any calculation here we make sure that we are adding quantities expressed in the same units (that is, both in litres, or both in millilitres). Since the answer is required in litres, we could start by writing both volumes in litres. So we are adding 1.5 litres and 0.145 litres. But using Strategy 2 above, this data could be converted to 1500 ml added to 145 ml, which we can probably do mentally: 1500 + 145 = 1645. The result, 1645 ml, can then be converted back to litres: 1.645 litres. Alternatively, setting out the calculation as a formal addition we would write 1.5 as 1.500 to ensure three digits after the decimal point in each number, like this:

$$1.5\,0\,0$$

$$+\ \underline{0.1\,4\,5}$$

$$1.6\,4\,5$$

What about multiplying a decimal number by a whole number?

In this section we consider examples of multiplications involving decimal numbers that you should expect to be able to do mentally. These would be examples where you would be able to do the calculation fairly easily if you removed the decimal point. For example you should be able to calculate 0.08×4 mentally, because (we hope!) you can already do $8 \times 4 (= 32)$.

We will first give you a standard way of dealing with multiplications involving decimals.

We can look at 0.08×4 and imagine there's no decimal point; think of the calculation as 008×4, which is the same as 8×4, which is 32. Now put the decimal point back!

Where do you put it? Well to change 0.08 to 8, you multiply by 100, so the answer 32 is 100 times too large. It must therefore be divided by 100, which moves the decimal point 2 places to the left, giving the answer 0.32.

Multiplying a decimal number by a whole number

Step 1: remove the decimal point

Step 2: do the multiplication with whole numbers

Step 3: put the decimal point back in the answer – make sure there are now as many digits after the decimal point as there were before you removed it!

From this example, we can see that because there were two digits after the decimal point in the decimal number being multiplied by a whole number there will be two digits after the decimal point in the answer. The same applies to any number of digits after the decimal point, of course.

In using this approach, make sure you don't throw away any zeros at the end of your answer before you put the decimal point back! Consider, for example, 0.012×5. We see this mentally, without the decimal point, as 12×5, which is 60. Now put the decimal point back, noting that to start with there were three digits after the point in 0.012, so we need three digits after the point in the answer. So the answer must be 0.060. Now it is safe, if appropriate, to drop the trailing zero, to give the result 0.06.

Example: 0.04 × 9

Step 1: change to 4×9

Step 2: $4 \times 9 = 36$

Step 3: we need to get back to two digits after the decimal point, so $0.04 \times 9 = 0.36$

EXAMPLE 9.6

In Spot the errors Statement 5 the calculation required is to multiply 0.04 by 6. Think of this as $4 \times 6 = 24$. Now put back the decimal point so there are once again two digits after it: $0.04 \times 6 = 0.24$.

EXAMPLE 9.7

In Spot the errors Statement 8 the calculation required is 4×0.225. Remove the decimal point for a moment and the calculation is 4×225. Do this by whatever method suits you. For example, you can always multiply by 4 by doubling and

(Continued)

(Continued)

doubling again. So double 225 is 450, and double 450 is 900. Now put the decimal point back to restore the three digits after the point, giving $4 \times 0.225 = 0.900$. The result is 0.900 g (which can also be written as 0.9 g).

EXAMPLE 9.8

In Spot the errors Statement 6 the calculation required is 25×1.8. So, start with 25×18, and do this multiplication by whatever method you are confident with. For example, we could think of eighteen 25s as twenty 25s subtract two 25s, which is $500 - 50 = 450$. Or you could think of it as $(25 \times 10) + (25 \times 8) = 250 + 200 = 450$.

Or you could do it using the grid method, as explained in Chapter 3. However you do it, you should get to $25 \times 18 = 450$. Now put the decimal point back, so that there is one digit following it, as there was before we removed it: $25 \times 1.8 = 45.0$. So the dose required is 45.0 mg (or just 45 mg).

How do you multiply together two decimal numbers?

Multiplying two decimal numbers

Step 1: remove the decimal points from both numbers

Step 2: do the multiplication with whole numbers

Step 3: put the decimal point back in the answer – make sure there are now as many digits after the decimal point as there were altogether in the two numbers before you removed their decimal points!

Say we had to find 0.7×0.125. If we drop the decimal point from the first number the calculation becomes 7×0.125. When we get the answer to this we would have to remember to put back the decimal point with one more digit after it. If we now drop the decimal point from the second number the calculation becomes 7×125. When we get the answer to this we have to reinstate a further three digits after the decimal point! So altogether we have four decimal places to put back in the answer to 7×125 to get the answer to 0.7×0.125. We then calculate 7×125 by an appropriate method, to get the result $7 \times 125 = 875$. Now get back to the four digits after the decimal point and we get: $0.7 \times 0.125 = 0.0875$.

We can explain this process by thinking in terms of repeatedly multiplying the numbers by 10 until we have whole numbers, and then undoing this by repeatedly dividing by 10. Remember that multiplying by 10 moves the decimal point one place to the right, and dividing by 10 moves it one place to the left.

We start with: 0.7×0.125

Multiply the first number by 10 and we get: 7×0.125

Multiply the second number by 10 and we get:	7×1.25
Multiply the second number by 10 again:	7×12.5
Multiply the second number by 10 again:	7×125

We now have a multiplication with whole numbers: $7 \times 125 = 875$

But to get to this we have multiplied by 10 four times, so we must now divide the result (875) by 10 four times:

Divide 875 by 10:	87.5
Divide it by 10 again:	8.75
Divide it by 10 again:	0.875
Divide it by 10 again:	0.0875

So, $0.7 \times 0.125 = 0.0875$.

EXAMPLE 9.9

The maximum total daily dose of oral paracetamol recommended for a neonate is 0.06 g per kilogram of weight. What would this be for a neonate weighing 2.4 kg?

The calculation required is 2.4×0.06. Dropping the decimal points this becomes $24 \times 6 = 144$. In dropping the decimal points we lose one digit after the decimal point in the 2.4 and two in the 0.06 – three in total. We must now reinstate these three digits after the decimal point in the 144, giving us $2.4 \times 0.06 = 0.144$. The maximum total daily dose is therefore 0.144 g (or 144 mg).

EXAMPLE 9.10

Drug G is prescribed at a dose of 12.5 mg per square metre of body surface area. A patient has a body surface area of 1.7 square metres. What is the correct dose of Drug G for this patient?

The calculation required is 12.5×1.7. We will first calculate 125×17, remembering that we have one decimal place to reinstate for the first number and another one for the second number: that's two places altogether.

Using an appropriate method, we find that $125 \times 17 = 2125$.

So, knowing that $125 \times 17 = 2125$, we put back the two decimal places required and get our result: $12.5 \times 1.7 = 21.25$. The required dose is 21.25 mg.

In practice, it may be appropriate to round this to the nearest milligram, giving a dose of 21 mg.

EXAMPLE 9.11

The recommended daily dose of Drug H is 0.15 g per kg of weight. What is the recommended dose for a woman weighing 62.5 kg?

The calculation required is 62.5 × 0.15. Altogether there are three digits after the decimal points in this multiplication. So we do the multiplication 625 × 15 and then remember to reinstate the three digits after the decimal point at the end. Using an appropriate method for multiplication we find that 625 × 15 = 9375. So we deduce that 62.5 × 0.15 = 9.375. The dose required is 9.375 g.

In practice, it may be appropriate to round this to one decimal place, giving a dose of 9.4 g.

What other ways are there of dealing with multiplications involving decimals?

Tip 1 for multiplying with decimals

Get rid of some of the decimals by changing the units of measurement to smaller units (for example, mg instead of grams)

We will give you two helpful tips here. First, remember that you always have the option of getting rid of some of the decimal places involved in a multiplication by changing to smaller units. For instance, in Example 9.9, the daily dose of 0.06 g may be converted to 60 mg (see Chapter 6). The question then requires the calculation of 2.4 × 60 mg: so you now have to deal with only one decimal number, not two. Similarly in Example 9.11, the dose of 0.15 g per kg of weight can be converted to 150 mg. So the recommended dose for the woman in question is 62.5 × 150 mg, which you may find easier to deal with than 62.5 × 0.150 g.

Tip 2 for multiplying with decimals

Make creative use of factors. For example,

24 × 0.25 mg
= 6 × 4 × 0.25 mg
= 6 × 1 mg = 6 mg.

Second, make creative use of factors, as we proposed for multiplication with whole numbers in Chapter 3. For example, to calculate 2.4 × 60 (see preceding paragraph) split the 60 mentally into two factors, 10 × 6, then multiply the 2.4 first by the 10 (to get 24). We have changed 2.4 × 60 into 24 × 6. In healthcare contexts you often have to do multiplications involving decimal numbers ending in 5. As we noted in Chapter 3, whenever we see a 5 at the end of a decimal number we will try to multiply it by 2! For example, some drugs are in doses of 2.5 mg. If we had 12 doses of 2.5 mg we would need to calculate 12 × 2.5. Think of the 12 as 6 × 2, and this becomes 6 × 2 × 2.5, which is 6 × 5 (= 30).

EXAMPLE 9.12

Over the course of a week a child receives 20 doses of 0.25 mg of paracetamol suspension. How much is that altogether? The calculation required is 20 × 0.25.

Think of the 20 as 10×2 and first multiply the 0.25 by the 2:

$20 \times 0.25 = 10 \times 2 \times 0.25 = 10 \times 0.5 = 5$.

In total the child has received 5 mg.

What do I need to know about division involving decimals?

In Chapter 3 we saw that the answer to a division stays the same if you multiply (or divide) both numbers by the same things. For example, $12 \div 5$ is the same as $24 \div 10$ (doubling both numbers) or $1.2 \div 0.5$ (dividing each number by 10). We can use this idea for division calculations that involve decimals numbers, especially when the first number in the division is greater than the second. Try to find creative ways of using this idea to get whole numbers and to make the calculation as easy as possible. Multiplying both numbers by 10 is often a good start.

Making divisions with decimals easier

You can multiply (or divide) both numbers in a division by the same number and not change the answer. Doing this creatively can make the division much easier.

For example, for $8 \div 0.2$ multiply both numbers by 5 and it becomes $40 \div 1$.

EXAMPLE 9.13

How many doses of 0.2 mg are there in a vial containing a total of 5 mg of a drug? The calculation required is $5 \div 0.2$.

Multiply both numbers by 10 and the calculation becomes $50 \div 2$ (= 25). So, there are 25 doses available.

EXAMPLE 9.14

The maximum total dosage of ibuprofen for a patient over 12 years in 24 hours is given as 2.4 g. Ibuprofen is available in 0.4 g tablets. How many tablets may be given in a day? The calculation required is $2.4 \div 0.4$.

Multiply both numbers by 10 and the calculation becomes $24 \div 4$, which equals 6. So 6 tablets may be given in one day.

There are two further things to note from Example 9.14.

First, the tablet would probably be described as 400 mg, rather than 0.4 g. Before dividing the 2.4 g by 400 mg it is essential that we put them into the same units: both in grams or both in milligrams. For the purposes of illustration here we have put them both into grams (2.4 g and 0.4 g). We could have put them both into milligrams (2400 mg and 400 mg) and the division would not have involved any decimals: $2400 \div 400 = 6$.

Dividing by a number less than 1

Notice in examples 9.13, 9.14 and 9.15 that when you divide a number N by a number less than 1 you get an answer *greater* than N. This is always the case. For example, 6 ÷ 0.4 will give an answer larger than 6.

Second, notice that when 2.4 is divided by 0.4 the answer is greater than 2.4. This is a general principle: if you divide by a number less than 1 then the answer you get will be greater than the number you started with. Some very common examples of this principle would be in simple calculations such as these: 5 ÷ 0.1 = 50; 10 ÷ 0.5 = 20; 3 ÷ 0.25 = 12. In each case, the reader should notice that the answer is greater than the number we start with, because it is being divided by something less than 1. Note also that the smaller the 'divisor' (the number you are dividing by), the greater the answer. Look at the results of these divisions, for example: 2 ÷ 1 = 2; 2 ÷ 0.1 = 20; 2 ÷ 0.01 = 200; 2 ÷ 0.001 = 2000, and so on.

EXAMPLE 9.15

The volume of each drop in a standard giving set (see Chapter 12) is 0.05 ml. How many drops are there in 62.5 ml? The calculation required is 62.5 ÷ 0.05.

Multiply both numbers by 100 to get a calculation without any decimals: 6250 ÷ 5 = 1250. So there are altogether 1250 drops in 62.5 ml.
(Here's another suggestion. Double each number, so 62.5 ÷ 0.05 becomes 125 ÷ 0.1. Now multiply both numbers by 10, to get 1250 ÷ 1, which equals 1250. Neat, eh?)

Divisions of a decimal number by a whole number will require the application of the short division procedure explained in Chapter 3. For example, Figure 9.2 shows the division of 11.25 by 6. This might be the calculation required if, say, a total dosage of 11.25 units has to be divided into 6 equal parts. We will explain the calculation in Figure 9.2 step by step.

(a) 6) 1 1.2 5

(b) 6) 1 1^5.2 5   1.

(c) 6) 1 1^5.2^{4}5   1.8

(d) 6) 1 1^5.2^{4}5^{3}0   1.8 7

(e) 6) 1 1^5.2^{4}5^{3}0   1.8 7 5

Figure 9.2 Dividing 11.25 by 6

Step (a): the calculation is set up in order to divide the 6 into the 11.25; the decimal point is inserted ready to receive the digits in the right places.

Step (b): 11 divided by 6 is 1, remainder 5; the 1 is placed in the units position above the line; the little 5 indicates that we 'carry' this remainder into the next column where it becomes 50, so we now have 52 in that column.

Step (c): 52 divided by 6 is 8, remainder 4; the 8 is put in the next position in the answer above the line; the 4 is carried to the next column where it becomes 40, so we now have 45 in that column.

Step (d): 45 divided by 6 is 7, remainder 3; the 7 is put in the answer above the line; the 3 must be carried to the next column, where currently there is not anything, so we insert a zero and attach the 3 to that; we now have 30 in that column.

Step (e): 30 divided by 6 is 5; the 5 is written in the answer. The calculation is complete: $11.25 \div 6 = 1.875$.

EXAMPLE 9.16

A volume of 1.25 litres is to be infused over a period of 8 hours. To find the volume to be infused each hour we need to calculate $1.25 \div 8$. The calculation is shown in Figure 9.3(a). The result is 0.15625 litres. Note that in order to complete this we had to write in three additional zeros so the calculation became $1.25000 \div 8$. The division begins: 12 divided by 8 is 1, remainder 4; carry the 4 to the next column, where we now have 45 … and so on.

Figure 9.3(b) shows what this calculation would have looked like if we had first converted the volume to 1250 millilitres. Then we would calculate $1250 \div 8$ and obtain the answer 156.25 ml. Yes, it would have looked exactly the same except for the position of the decimal point!

In practice these results would probably be rounded. To three significant digits they are 0.156 litres, or 156 ml, giving an infusion rate of 156 ml per hour.

$$\text{(a)} \quad 8\,\overline{)\,1.2^4 5^5 0^2 0^4 0\,} = 0.15625$$

$$\text{(b)} \quad 8\,\overline{)\,1\,2^4 5^5 0.^2 0^4 0\,} = 156.25$$

Figure 9.3 Comparing $1.25 \div 8$ and $1250 \div 8$

Any division calculations that are more demanding than the examples in this section would best be done on a calculator.

Checking that the result of a calculation involving decimals is reasonable

Round each number to one significant digit (or at most 2 significant digits) and find their product.

This approximate answer should at least give an indication of whether or not you have the decimal point in the right place.

How do I check the reasonableness of the answer to a multiplication or division involving decimal numbers?

You can check that the answer to a calculation involving decimal numbers is reasonable by rounding each number to one (or at the most two) significant digits (see Chapter 8) and using these to get an approximation to the correct result. You should be able to do this mentally, using the principles explained in the preceding sections. The result should indicate to you whether or not you have got the decimal point in the right place – which is the most likely error you might make.

EXAMPLE 9.17

In Example 9.7, the calculation required was 4×0.225. Rounding to one significant digit this becomes 4×0.2, which equals 0.8. This indicates that the answer of 0.9 is about right and that we have not made an error in placing the decimal point.

EXAMPLE 9.18

In Example 9.8 the calculation required was 25×1.8. Rounding the 1.8 to one significant digit this becomes 25×2, which is equal to 50. This indicates that the answer of 45 is about right and that we have not made an error in placing the decimal point.

EXAMPLE 9.19

Drug J is prescribed for an infant at a dosage of 0.36 g per kilogram of weight. The dosage for an infant weighing 3.2 kg is calculated by multiplying 0.36 by 3.2. A nurse calculates that the dose should be 0.1152 g. Is this reasonable?

Rounding the numbers to one significant digit the calculation becomes 0.4×3, which equals 1.2. We should expect the answer to be around 1.2 g, suggesting that 0.1152 g has the decimal point in the wrong place. (The correct result is 1.152 g.)

> ## EXAMPLE 9.20
>
> In Example 9.16 we found that 1.25 ÷ 8 was equal to 0.15625. Does this answer look reasonable? Rounding the 1.25 to 1 gives us 1 ÷ 8. In Chapter 11 we will explain how 1 ÷ 8 is equal to the fraction ⅛ and how this is equal to 0.125. If we know this, then we have a clear indication that 0.15625 looks like a reasonable answer – at least the decimal point looks as though it is in the right place.

You should not need to use a calculator for any of these check-up questions.

9.1 Practise your addition and subtraction of decimal numbers by completing the grid in Figure 9.4. As you move from one cell to the next, left to right along the rows, add 0.4; as you move from one cell to the next down the columns subtract 0.07. If you do it all correctly you will get to 1.62 in the bottom right-hand corner.

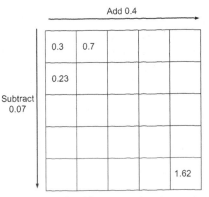

Figure 9.4 Grid for practice of addition and subtraction with decimals (check-up question 9.1)

9.2 Practise your multiplication and division with decimal numbers by completing the multiplication table in Figure 9.5.

×	0.02	0.05	0.4		0.8
5				2.5	
					1.6
0.5			0.2		
0.2					
0.1		0.005			

Figure 9.5 Multiplication grid with decimal numbers (check-up question 9.2)

(Continued)

(Continued)

The number in each cell within the table is obtained by multiplying together the numbers in the headings for the row and column in which that cell lies. For example, the 0.2 in the centre of the table is the product of 0.4 and 0.5.

9.3   Double these doses:

(a) 0.5 ml   (b) 0.25 mg

(c) 1.5 g   (d) 0.125 mg

9.4   Multiply these doses by 4:

(a) 0.5 micrograms   (b) 0.25 g

(c) 1.25 mg   (d) 0.125 litres

9.5   A patient with pulmonary oedema is receiving an intravenous infusion that contains 0.2 mg of GTN in each ml. The infusion is set to deliver 20 ml each hour. What dosage of GTN is contained in this 20 ml? (The calculation required is 20×0.2.)

9.6   A patient is prescribed a dobutamine preparation to be delivered by intravenous infusion at the rate of 2.5 micrograms per minute for each kilogram of the patient's body weight. What is the dose required per minute if the patient's body weight is 72 kg? (The calculation required is 2.5×72.)

9.7   Dobutamine is available as a stock item in a 20-ml ampoule containing 12.5 mg per ml. What is the total amount in milligrams of dobutamine in the 20-ml ampoule? (The calculation required is 20×12.5.)

9.8   How many 0.4 mg doses of Drug K are required to give a total dose of 20 mg?

9.9   How many 0.04 mg doses of Drug L are required to give a total dose of 2 mg?

9.10   Use rounding to check if these results are reasonable or if they look like they might contain an error in the position of the decimal point:

(a) $0.0325 \times 8 = 0.26$

(b) $23.8 \times 0.075 = 17.85$

(c) $12.5 \div 0.0475 = 263$ (to 3 significant digits)

(d) $0.085 \div 0.28 = 0.00304$ (to 3 significant digits)

IMPERIAL UNITS STILL IN USE

10

OBJECTIVES

In a practical healthcare context the practitioner should be able to:

- know rough equivalences in metric units of imperial units of length, weight and liquid volume still commonly used by patients
- convert between metric units of length and imperial units still used in particular contexts
- convert between metric units of weight and imperial units still met in particular contexts
- convert between litres and imperial units of liquid volume still met in particular contexts

SPOT THE ERRORS

Identify any obvious errors in converting between imperial and metric units in the following six statements.

1   An adult patient gives their height as 5 foot 10 inches. A practice nurse uses a conversion chart to convert this to 1.78 m.

2   A metre is about 25.4 inches.

3   The weight of a newborn baby boy is reported by his mother to be 6 lb 10 oz. This is equivalent to about 3 kg.

4   The length of a newborn baby girl is reported by her mother to be 19.7 inches. This is equivalent to about 500 mm.

5   A weight of 11 stone is equivalent to about 70 kg.

6   A litre of fluid is just over half a pint.

Are the errors you have spotted potentially serious in medical health practice?

(errors identified on page 118)

Is knowledge of imperial units needed in healthcare practice?

This chapter should not be necessary. The use of metric units for measuring length, weight and liquid volume are now standard in all professional practice and most commercial activity in the UK. But a number of so-called imperial units survive in everyday life and make their way informally into healthcare situations.

We should really expect to see lengths expressed in kilometres, metres, centimetres, millimetres, and so on. Yet all the distances on our road signs are still expressed in miles (a non-metric, imperial unit). A warning sign might contain both imperial yards and metric metres, as in this one: '200 yards ahead, low bridge, maximum height 4 metres'. Most people still give their height in feet and inches, with 'six feet' regarded as the point at which a man is regarded as tall.

We should likewise expect to see all measurements of weight (or mass) in kilograms, grams, milligrams and so on. But the stallholders in Norwich Market, for example, have resisted all EU attempts to get them to price their fruit and vegetables by the kilogram and continue to sell their produce by the pound (weight). Few people seem to know their own body weight in kilograms. And the proud parents will almost always disregard the metric version of their new baby's weight and choose to report it to their family and friends as, say, 7 pounds 10 ounces (rather than 3.46 kg).

In terms of liquid volume, the metric units of litres and millilitres are fairly widespread in real-life contexts, but you might still get a pint of ale at your local hostelry, and some milk is still sold in pints. And why do so many people – all of whom buy their petrol in litres – insist on telling us how many miles their car does to the *gallon*?

The point we are making is that we in the UK live in a society that uses a potentially confusing mix of imperial and metric units. It is therefore important for clear communication that healthcare practitioners are at least able to help their patients make sense of the measurements we share with them. We are also aware of the fact that younger adults entering healthcare practice may be relatively unfamiliar with imperial units, having been taught in schools only how to work in metric. It is on this basis that we have specified the objectives for this chapter. To achieve these objectives we suggest that you need four things: knowledge of how the most frequently-used imperial units relate to each other; the ability to use conversion tables and charts; memorization of some useful reference items; the use of conversion factors.

What relationships between imperial units should be known?

In measurements of length, the only imperial units likely to turn up in a healthcare context are *feet* and *inches*. A foot is about the length of one of Derek's shoes and an

ERRORS IDENTIFIED

The obvious errors are Statements 2 and 6.

Statement 2

The person making this statement may be misremembering this conversion: 1 inch equals 25.4 mm (or 2.54 cm). A metre is actually about 39.4 inches.

Statement 6

The person making this statement may be confusing it with the correct assertion that a pint of fluid is just over half a litre. To three significant digits, a pint is equal to 0.568 litres. This gives a litre as about 1.76 pints (roughly a pint and three-quarters).

These errors are unlikely to be serious in a healthcare context, since for clinical purposes all measurements should be made using metric units. However, it is often helpful for good practitioner–patient communication if the practitioner is able with some confidence to make conversions between imperial units still in common use and the metric units used by professionals.

(now continue reading from page 117)

Archaic units, but still alive and active

1 foot = 12 inches
1 stone = 14 pounds
1 pound = 16 ounces

inch is about the width of his thumb – but then he does have quite large feet and hands. You need to know that there are 12 inches in a foot. So, for example, the height of a woman given as 5 feet 6 inches can also be given as 66 inches [(5 × 12) + 6 = 66]; and the height of a child given as 3 feet 7 inches could also be given as 43 inches [(3 × 12) + 7 = 43]. The abbreviation for 3 feet and 7 inches is usually *3 ft 7 ins,* but you may also encounter 3′ 7″.

In measurements of weight, we have to be familiar with stones and pounds (for adult body weight) and pounds and ounces (for neonate body weight). Many overweight people would like to lose about a stone in weight and refer to the extra weight around their midriff as their 'spare tyre'. This is a helpful image, since a stone is about the weight of a tyre on a small car. A pound is the weight of about four medium-sized apples. And an ounce is about the weight of a small packet of crisps. The relationships between these units seem very archaic: 14 pounds = 1 stone, and 16 ounces = 1 pound; likewise the abbreviations: *lb* for pound (from the Latin word *libra*), and *oz* for ounce (from an old Italian word, *onza*). So, for example, a body weight of 11 stone 6 lb is equivalent to 160 lb [(11 × 14) + 6 = 160]. And a neonate's weight of 6 lb 4 oz is equivalent to 100 oz [(6 × 16) + 4 = 100].

The only imperial unit of liquid volume that might just turn up occasionally in an informal healthcare context is the pint, so we do not need to know how this relates to other imperial units of liquid volume, such as the gallon or the fluid ounce.

What we do need to know, however, is how these imperial units relate to the metric units that are invariably used in professional practice. A conversion table or chart is one way of accessing this relationship.

What are conversion tables and charts?

In a conversion table, measurements in imperial units are placed alongside or above or below their equivalent measurements in a metric unit. Figure 10.1 is a conversion table for feet and inches to metres, which would be useful for interpreting a patient's height given to you in imperial units. Each measurement in feet and inches has its metric equivalent immediately below it.

4 ft 0 ins	4 ft 1 ins	4 ft 2 ins	4 ft 3 ins	4 ft 4 ins	4 ft 5 ins
1.22 m	1.24 m	1.27 m	1.30 m	1.32 m	1.35 m
4 ft 6 ins	4 ft 7 ins	4 ft 8 ins	4 ft 9 ins	4 ft 10 ins	4 ft 11 ins
1.37 m	1.40 m	1.42 m	1.45 m	1.47 m	1.50 m
5 ft 0 ins	5 ft 1 ins	5 ft 2 ins	5 ft 3 ins	5 ft 4 ins	5 ft 5 ins
1.52 m	1.55 m	1.57 m	1.60 m	1.63 m	1.65 m
5 ft 6 ins	5 ft 7 ins	5 ft 8 ins	5 ft 9 ins	5 ft 10 ins	5 ft 11 ins
1.68 m	1.70 m	1.73 m	1.75 m	1.78 m	1.80 m
6 ft 0 ins	6 ft 1 ins	6 ft 2 ins	6 ft 3 ins	6 ft 4 ins	6 ft 5 ins
1.83 m	1.85 m	1.88 m	1.91 m	1.93 m	1.96 m
6 ft 6 ins	6 ft 7 ins	6 ft 8 ins	6 ft 9 ins	6 ft 10 ins	6 ft 11 ins
1.98 m	2.01 m	2.03 m	2.06 m	2.08 m	2.11 m

Figure 10.1   Conversion table for feet and inches to metres

This table covers heights from 4 feet to 6 feet 11 inches, which is a range of heights within which nearly all UK adults would fall. The heights in metres are rounded (see Chapter 8) to three significant digits (or, in this case, to two decimal places or the nearest centimetre).

EXAMPLE 10.1

Use the conversion table in Figure 10.1 to check the conversion referred to in Spot the errors Statement 1.

The height of 5 ft 10 ins is located in the table. The entry in metres below it shows this to be equivalent to 1.78 m.

Figure 10.2 is a similar table that could be used for converting the length of a neonate in centimetres to a length in inches – units that might be more familiar to some parents. The lengths in inches are given to three significant digits (or, in this case, to one decimal place or the nearest tenth of an inch). The range of lengths given here is from 30 to 59 centimetres; the body lengths of most neonates lie between 35 and 51 cm.

30 cm	31 cm	32 cm	33 cm	34 cm
11.8 ins	12.2 ins	12.6 ins	13.0 ins	13.4 ins
35 cm	36 cm	37 cm	38 cm	39 cm
13.8 ins	14.2 ins	14.6 ins	15.0 ins	15.4 ins
40 cm	41 cm	42 cm	43 cm	44 cm
15.7 ins	16.1 ins	16.5 ins	16.9 ins	17.3 ins
45 cm	46 cm	47 cm	48 cm	49 cm
17.7 ins	18.1 ins	18.5 ins	18.9 ins	19.3 ins
50 cm	51 cm	52 cm	53 cm	54 cm
19.7 ins	20.1 ins	20.5 ins	20.9 ins	21.3 ins
55 cm	56 cm	57 cm	58 cm	59 cm
21.7 ins	22.0 ins	22.4 ins	22.8 ins	23.2 ins

Figure 10.2   Conversion table for centimetres to inches

EXAMPLE 10.2

Use the conversion table in Figure 10.2 to check the conversion referred to in Spot the errors Statement 4.

A length of 500 mm is the same as 50 cm. This measurement is located in the table. The entry in inches below 50 cm shows that it is equivalent to 19.7 inches (to 3 significant digits).

Figure 10.3 is a similar conversion table for converting the weight of a neonate or young child from kilograms (rounded to one decimal place) to ounces (rounded to the nearest ounce). This provides conversion data for weights in the range 2.0 kg to 4.9 kg, which would include the birth-weights of almost all non-premature babies in the U.K

2.0 kg	2.1 kg	2.2 kg	2.3 kg	2.4 kg
71 oz	74 oz	78 oz	81 oz	85 oz
2.5 kg	2.6 kg	2.7 kg	2.8 kg	2.9 kg
88 oz	92 oz	95 oz	99 oz	102 oz
3.0 kg	3.1 kg	3.2 kg	3.3 kg	3.4 kg
106 oz	109 oz	113 oz	116 oz	120 oz
3.5 kg	3.6 kg	3.7 kg	3.8 kg	3.9 kg
123 oz	127 oz	131 oz	134 oz	138 oz
4.0 kg	4.1 kg	4.2 kg	4.3 kg	4.4 kg
141 oz	145 oz	148 oz	152 oz	155 oz
4.5 kg	4.6 kg	4.7 kg	4.8 kg	4.9 kg
159 oz	162 oz	166 oz	169 oz	173 oz

Figure 10.3 Conversion table for kilograms to ounces

EXAMPLE 10.3

Check the conversion referred to in Spot the errors Statement 3

The weight of 3.0 kg is located in the table. Immediately below this is the equivalent weight in ounces: 106 oz, to the nearest ounce. Since there are 16 ounces in a pound and $6 \times 16 = 96$, then 106 oz = 6 lb 10 oz.

A similar conversion table to that shown in Figure 10.3 could be used for adult weights. Figure 10.4 shows another convenient way of doing conversions between units, using a graphical representation. This conversion chart is for converting an adult patient's weight in stones and pounds to the equivalent weight in kilograms. It does not provide such detailed information as the tables in Figures 10.1–3, but the context in which such a conversion might be done does not usually require a high level of precision. To make a conversion you just read directly from one scale to the other. For example, we can see that 15 stone is just a bit over 95 kg (it is actually 95.25 kg to two decimal places). Similarly we can see that 120 kg is just short of 19 stone (it is actually 18 stone 13 pounds, to the nearest pound). This level of accuracy is quite sufficient for answering the patient's question, 'what is that in old money?' when they are told their weight in kilograms.

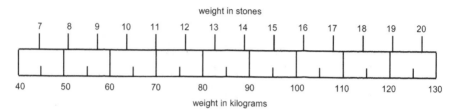

Figure 10.4   Linear conversion chart for weights in stones and kilograms

Figure 10.5 shows another chart representing the relationship between metric and imperial units in a graphical format. The arrows show how this can be used to read off a weight in pounds (lb) in kilograms (kg), or vice versa. This particular chart covers weights from 0 kg to 30 kg and could be used, for example, for approximate conversions for the weights of children up to the age of three years. The arrows show: (a) how a weight of 44 lb on the vertical axis is matched via a point on the graph to the equivalent weight in kilograms on the horizontal axis (20 kg); and (b) how a weight of 10 kg on the horizontal axis is matched via a point on the graph to the equivalent weight in pounds on the vertical axis (22 lb).

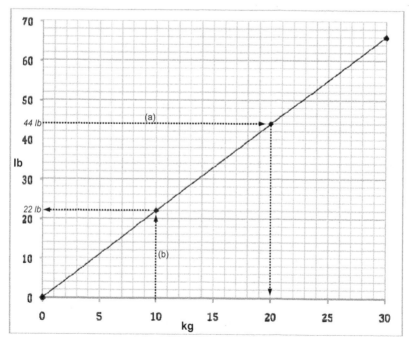

Figure 10.5   Conversion graph for kilograms and pounds

EXAMPLE 10.4

(a) A practice nurse measures an adult patient's weight as 86 g. The patient asks what this is in stones. In Figure 10.4 the weight of 86 g is on the lower scale just beyond the mark for 85 kg that is halfway between 80 kg and 90 kg. The point above this on the top scale gives the equivalent weight as about 13 stone 7 lb.

(b) A child aged 4 years weighs 22 kg. A paediatrician wants a rough conversion to pounds for the benefit of the mother. Using the graph in Figure 10.5, the weight of 22 kg is located on the horizontal axis. Follow the vertical line from this point on the scale up to the diagonal line (straight line graph), then follow a horizontal line to the vertical axis. Read off the corresponding weight in pounds, as just over 48 lb (which is 3 stone 6 lb).

What reference items might be memorized?

It is helpful to be able to recall instantly some particular conversions between imperial and metric, so that you can relate other measurements to these. These are your personal reference items.

Reference items for conversions of length

- Memorize your own height in metric and imperial
- Memorize one other height conversion, such as 4 ft 11 ins = 1.5 m.
- Remember that 12 inches (a foot) is about 30 cm.

For measurements of adult height you might start by remembering your own height both in metres and in feet and inches. Paul, for example, knows that he is 1.80 m tall, and that this is equivalent to about 5 ft 11 ins. Then pick one other height some way away from your own and memorize that. For example, Paul always remembers that 4 ft 11 ins (59 inches) is 1.5 m (one and a half metres).

Also, remember that a standard ruler with both metric and imperial scales will be a 12-inch (one foot) ruler on one scale and a 30-cm (or 300 mm) ruler on the other. So, 10 cm is about 4 inches. And that means that 100 cm (a metre) is about 40 inches (39.4 inches is a more accurate conversion: see *Spot the errors* Statement 2 and its correction.)

EXAMPLE 10.5

Use that fact that a length of 30 cm is about 12 inches to convert a neonate's length of 45 cm to inches (approximately). Check this against the conversion given in Figure 10.2.

If 30 cm is about 12 ins, then 15 cm is about 6 ins. Adding these, 45 cm is about 18 ins. Figure 10.2 gives 45 cm more accurately as 17.7 ins, which is 18 ins to the nearest inch.

Reference items for conversions of weight

Memorize your own weight in metric and imperial

11 stone is about 70 kg

15 stone is about 95 kg

A birth weight of 3.4 kg is about 7 lb 8 oz

Introducing proportionality (more in Chapter 12)

If two variables are (directly) proportional to each other then:

(a) to get from a value of one variable to the corresponding value of the other you always multiply by the same factor;

(b) when the value of one variable is multiplied (or divided) by some number the corresponding value of the other variable is multiplied (or divided) by the same number;

(c) when one is zero the other is zero;

(d) the relationship between them can be represented by a straight line graph passing through the origin.

Conversion factors, metric to imperial

To 3 significant digits:

1 m = 39.4 inches

1 cm = 0.394 inches

1 kg = 2.20 pounds

1 g = 0.0353 ounces

1 litre = 1.76 pints

In the same way, know your own weight in both metric and imperial, and memorize at least one other (such as 15 stone is about 95 kg). A useful reference point is 11 stone. Figure 10.4 shows that this lands almost bang on 70 kg. Then learn at least one birth weight (it could be your own or a baby known to you) in both metric and imperial. For example, a fairly average birth weight of 3.4 kg is about seven and a half pounds (7 lb 8 oz).

How do conversion factors work?

A measurement made on a metric scale and the equivalent measurement in an imperial unit are two *variables* that are *proportional* to each other (strictly speaking they are *directly* proportional). Proportionality is one of the most important ideas in mathematics, and one that we will explain in more detail in Chapter 12. What it means effectively is that the two variables are related to each other in such a way that the value of one is always a constant factor multiplied by the other.

Here is a very simple everyday example: if apples are priced at £1.65 per kilogram, then there are two variables involved in a purchase of apples: (a) the weight of apples in kilograms, and (b) the cost of the purchase in pounds. And the relationship between these variables (allowing for any rounding required) is that the cost in £ is always 1.65 multiplied by the weight in kg, whatever weight is selected. So, if we purchase 2.4 kg of apples, the cost will be £1.65 × 2.4 (= £3.96). If we purchase 0.8 kg, then the cost will be £1.65 × 0.8 (= £1.32).

It is the same with measurements in metric and imperial units, when the number you multiply by is called the *conversion factor*.

So a measurement of a length made in inches is proportional to the same measurement made in centimetres. The conversion factor is just the number of centimetres in an inch, which is 2.54 (incidentally, this is an exact value, because an inch is defined as 2.54 centimetres). So to convert a length in centimetres to inches we just multiply by 2.54. For example, 72 inches is 72 × 2.54 cm = 182.88 cm.

Similarly, the conversion factor for relating measurements of weight in stones to kilograms is the number of kilograms in a stone, which is 6.35 kg (to 3 significant digits). So to convert stones to kilograms we just multiply by 6.35. For example, 11 stone is 11 × 6.35 kg = 69.85 kg.

For converting pints to litres, the conversion factor (to 3 significant digits) is 0.568, since 1 pint = 0.568 litres. So, to convert pints to litres we multiply by 0.568. For example, half a pint (0.5 pints) is equal to 0.5 × 0.568 litres = 0.284 litres (or 284 ml).

We give two lists of conversion factors for reference. No one will expect you to memorize all these. Refer to these when needed and just make sure you know how to use them.

Notice also that when two variables are proportional then if you double one, you double the other; if you halve one, you halve the other. If you multiply one by 3, you multiply the other by 3, and so on. For example, if I know that 11 stone = 70 kg (approximately), then I can halve both values and deduce that 5.5 stone = 35 kg. If I know that 0.5 pints = 0.284 litres, then, multiplying both by 10, I know that 5 pints = 2.84 litres. We will exploit this property of proportionality in many kinds of healthcare calculations in Chapters 12–15.

Conversion factors, imperial to metric

1 inch = 2.54 cm (exact)

To 3 significant digits:

1 foot = 0.305 m

1 stone = 6.35 kg

1 pound = 454 g

1 ounce = 28.3 g

1 pint = 0.568 litres

There are two further important observations about proportionality. First, if two variables are proportional then corresponding values are matched to each other by a straight-line graph, like the one shown in Figure 10.5. Second, notice that this graph passes through the point where the two axes meet (this is called the *origin*). This is because two variables can only be proportional if when one variable takes the value zero then so does the other one. For example, 0 cm = 0 inches; 0 kg = 0 lb; 0 litres = 0 pints; and no apples cost nothing! By contrast, consider the two scales (Fahrenheit and Celsius) for measuring temperatures. These are *not* proportional. We know this because 0 °C does not equal 0 °F. (In fact 0 °C = 32 °F.) So, you cannot change a Celsius temperature to a Fahrenheit temperature (or vice versa) just by multiplying by a constant factor.

EXAMPLE 10.6

Use a calculator and the appropriate conversion factors to convert (a) 12.3 kg to pounds; (b) 0.75 of a pint to litres; (c) 3.5 ounces to grams; (d) 1.9 metres to inches. Give answers to 2 significant digits.

Answers: (a) 27 lb (12.3 × 2.20 = 27.06); (b) 0.43 litres (0.75 × 0.568 = 0.426); (c) 99 g (3.5 × 28.3 = 99.05); (d) 75 ins (1.9 × 39.4 = 74.86).

In this chapter we may have given more attention than might seem necessary to the imperial units used in everyday life, but not used in measurements in healthcare practice. However, we hope that on the way the reader will have done some useful and sophisticated mathematical thinking!

10.1   Use any of the methods given in this chapter to rewrite the following para-graph using imperial units, with measurements given to the nearest ounce.

The average birth weight of a baby born in the UK is 3.3 kg but weight can vary widely, between about 2.5 kg and 5 kg with girls tending to be around 300 g lighter than boys.

10.2   Now rewrite this paragraph with measurements in centimetres, rounded to two significant digits.

The average length of newborn babies in the UK is around 18 to 22 inches. They should normally grow about 1 to 1.5 inches in length during the first month.

10.3   Which is greater?

(a) 2 metres or 6 feet?   (b) 1 litre or 2 pints?

(c) 10 cm or 6 inches?   (d) 10 stone or 50 kg?

(e) 250 g or half a pound?

10.4   From the table in Figure 10.3 we can read off that a weight of 2.0 kg is equiva-lent to 71 ounces. Why is a weight of 4.0 kg not double this (142 ounces)?

10.5   Use the data provided in Figure 10.3 to complete the table Figure 10.6. This con-tains the same measurements as in Figure 10.3, but the imperial measurements are to be given in pounds and ounces, rather than just in ounces. To get you started, some conversions are already entered. Reminder: there are 16 ounces in a pound.

2.0 kg	2.1 kg	2.2 kg	2.3 kg	2.4 kg
4 lb 7 oz				
2.5 kg	2.6 kg	2.7 kg	2.8 kg	2.9 kg
	5 lb 12 oz			
3.0 kg	3.1 kg	3.2 kg	3.3 kg	3.4 kg
		7 lb 1 oz		
3.5 kg	3.6 kg	3.7 kg	3.8 kg	3.9 kg
			8 lb 6 oz	
4.0 kg	4.1 kg	4.2 kg	4.3 kg	4.4 kg
				9 lb 11 oz
4.5 kg	4.6 kg	4.7 kg	4.8 kg	4.9 kg

Figure 10.6   Conversion table for kilograms to pounds and ounces

UNDERSTANDING FRACTIONS AND RATIOS 11

OBJECTIVES

In everyday and healthcare contexts the practitioner should be able to:

- interpret a fraction as a proportion of a whole unit or set
- recognize what must be added to a fraction to make 1
- interpret a fraction as the division of one number by another
- interpret a fraction as a ratio
- recognize equivalent fractions or equivalent ratios
- use cancelling to simplify a fraction or a ratio
- express a ratio as 'one to something' or 'something to one'
- use mixed numbers
- state common equivalences between fractions and decimal numbers
- convert a fraction into a decimal number, or vice versa
- calculate a simple fraction of a number or quantity using informal mental, written or calculator methods

In this chapter our focus is on explaining the different concepts and principles involved in handling quantities expressed in fraction notation. To do this we use a mixture of everyday examples and some simple but occasionally rather artificial healthcare illustrations. In some cases we use results that turn up in the middle of the kinds of drug and infusion calculations that are explained in full in Chapter 12. This is a long chapter, which for some readers may require persistence and concentration. But if you work hard at the content here you should emerge with a deeper understanding of some key concepts that will enable you to engage with the mathematical demands of healthcare practice with greater confidence.

SPOT THE ERRORS

Identify any obvious errors in the use of fraction notation in the following 15 statements.

1 If a bar of chocolate is divided into 4 equal pieces and 3 of them are eaten then the amount eaten is $\frac{3}{4}$ of the bar.

2 If 3 bars of chocolate are shared equally between 4 people then each gets $\frac{3}{4}$ of a bar.

3 A patient's dosage of Drug A is reduced from 4 mg to 3 mg each day. The new dose is $\frac{3}{4}$ of the original dose.

4 If 8 out of 10 nurses in a hospital are female then $\frac{4}{5}$ of them are female.

5 A patient's dosage of Drug B is reduced from 12 mg to 9 mg each day. The new dose is $\frac{9}{12}$ of the original dose, which is equivalent to $\frac{2}{3}$ of the dose.

6 If $\frac{3}{8}$ of the contents of a bottle of medicine remains then $\frac{5}{8}$ has been used.

7 If person A earns £12 an hour and person B earns £9 an hour then A's rate of pay is $1\frac{1}{3}$ times B's.

8 In Statement 7 the ratio of B's rate of pay to A's rate of pay is 3:4.

9 Three quarters of a millilitre is the same as 0.75 ml.

10 An infant gaining 0.4 kg in weight has gained $\frac{2}{5}$ of a kilogram.

11 If $\frac{5}{8}$ of a litre of a suspension has been infused then the volume that has been infused is 0.58 litres.

12 Two thirds of a litre expressed in decimal form is 0.667 litres to three significant digits.

13 A patient with pulmonary oedema is receiving 4 mg of GTN in an infusion each hour. This is equivalent to $\frac{4}{60}$ mg per minute, which is 0.15 mg per minute.

14 A dose of 0.025 mg is $\frac{1}{40}$ mg, so there are 40 of these doses in a milligram.

15 Two thirds of 480 mg is 320 mg and three quarters of 480 mg is 360 mg.

Are the errors you have spotted potentially serious in medical health practice?

(errors identified on page 130)

What is the meaning of fraction notation?

We assume the reader is familiar with simple fractions, like a half ($\frac{1}{2}$), a quarter ($\frac{1}{4}$), three quarters ($\frac{3}{4}$), a third ($\frac{1}{3}$), and so on. But many people do not realize that a fraction can mean at least three different things.

Consider the simple fraction $\frac{3}{5}$ (three fifths). The number on the top of the fraction is called the *numerator* and the number on the bottom is called the *denominator* – but we give you permission to call them the top and bottom numbers. The simplest meaning of this notation is that it represents a proportion of a whole unit or a set. It is what you get if you take something, divide it into equal parts, and then take some of these parts. The denominator tells you how many parts to divide it into and the numerator tells you how many parts you get. So '$\frac{3}{4}$ of an hour' means 'divide an hour into 4 equal parts (quarters of an hour) and take 3 of them'. Similarly, '$\frac{3}{5}$ of a pizza' would be what you get if you were to divide a pizza into 5 equal slices (each slice is a fifth of the pizza) and then take 3 slices, as shown in Figure 11.1.

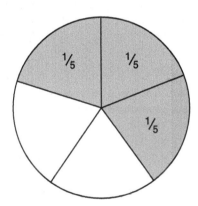

Figure 11.1   Three fifths ($\frac{3}{5}$) of a pizza

Note that the word 'proportion' is used here in a different sense from how it was used in Chapter 10. There it was used to describe a relationship between two variables. So we talked about two variables being *in proportion* to each other and one being *proportional* to the other. For example: 'The cost of apples bought is proportional to their weight'. Here we talk about *a proportion,* which just means a share of something, a portion, a part; in other words, a fraction. For example: 'A large proportion of people get confused by this word because it is used in these two different senses'.

Example 11.1 below illustrates that the thing that is divided up could be: (a) a single entity, such as a pizza or a chocolate bar; (b) a unit of measurement, such as a litre or a kilogram; (c) a set.

ERRORS IDENTIFIED

The obvious errors are Statements 5, 11, and 13.

Statement 5

It is correct to say that the dose of 9 mg is $^9/_{12}$ of the original dose of 12 mg. But this fraction is not equivalent to $^2/_3$. Dividing both the top number and the bottom number in $^9/_{12}$ by 3 ('cancelling' 3) simplifies this to the equivalent fraction $^3/_4$.

Statement 11

As we explain later in this chapter, the fraction $^5/_8$ expressed as a decimal is 0.625. So the volume that has been infused is 0.625 litres.

Statement 13

By cancelling 4, the fraction $^4/_{60}$ can be simplified to $^1/_{15}$. This fraction is *not* equal to 0.15. It is equal to '1 divided by 15', which gives 0.067 to three decimal places. The patient is receiving 0.067 mg per minute or 67 micrograms per minute.

The error in Statement 13 in particular is potentially serious. Although fractions are not generally used in clinical practice to express quantities – which are almost always expressed in decimal form – fractions will appear at times in the intermediate stages of dosage and infusion calculations and it is essential that these are correctly converted into decimal form. As we shall see in Chapter 12, having an understanding of fractions and ratios will help the practitioner to work out dosage and infusion rate calculations efficiently and correctly – as well as facilitating the equitable distribution of chocolate bars and pizzas.

(now continue reading from page 129)

EXAMPLE 11.1

What is the meaning of $^5/_8$ (five eighths)?

(a) You would get five eighths ($^5/_8$) of a sheet of paper by folding the sheet into 8 equal pieces and then cutting out a piece containing 5 of these.

(b) If a jug containing a litre of water is equivalent to 8 tumblers of water, then a patient drinking 5 of these tumblers has drunk five eighths ($^5/_8$) of a litre.

(c) If five eighths ($^5/_8$) of a supply of tablets are required, we could share the supply equally between 8 smaller boxes and then take 5 of these boxes.

When we take a fraction of a whole unit or a set, what is left behind is also a fraction. You should be able to state immediately what this is. For example, in Figure 11.1, if you take 3 of the slices ($^3/_5$ of the pizza) you leave 2 behind. So the fraction not taken is $^2/_5$ (two fifths). The whole pizza is 5 fifths ($^5/_5$) of a pizza. So $^5/_5 = 1$. And the $^3/_5$ added to the $^2/_5$ is the whole pizza: $^3/_5 + ^2/_5 = ^5/_5 = 1$.

The meaning of fractions

The fraction $^3/_5$ could mean:

- divide something or a set into 5 equal parts and take 3 of them;

- share 3 things equally between 5 (3 ÷ 5);

- the ratio of 3 to 5 (3:5)

Similarly in Example 11.1(b), if you use $^5/_8$ of a litre, then $^3/_8$ of a litre is not used. And $^5/_8$ of a litre + $^3/_8$ of a litre = $^8/_8$ of a litre = 1 litre.

This elementary idea of a fraction – as a proportion of a whole unit or of a set – is not the only meaning to be associated with the fraction notation. More importantly, we can also use a fraction like $^3/_5$ to represent a division or to represent a ratio.

How does a fraction represent a division?

The fraction $^3/_5$ can also mean: 'take 3 things and share them equally between 5'. In other words, $^3/_5$ also means '3 divided by 5'. So, for example, if we have 3 bars of chocolate and share them between 5 people, each person gets the equivalent of $^3/_5$ of a bar. This is illustrated in Figure 11.2.

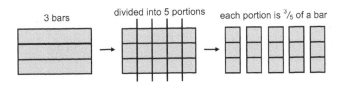

3 bars   divided into 5 portions   each portion is $^3/_5$ of a bar

Figure 11.2   The fraction $^3/_5$ seen as '3 divided by 5'

EXAMPLE 11.2

A total dosage of 5 g of Drug C is to be given in 8 equal doses. So each dose will be 5 g divided by 8, which is $^5/_8$ of a gram. (In practice this would then be expressed as a decimal, as explained later in this chapter. See also check-up question 11.8 at the end of the chapter.)

Fractions and division

Example: divide 3 by 4:

the calculation is 3 ÷ 4

this is also written 3/4

and the result is $^3/_4$

The really clever thing here is that $^5/_8$ is both an instruction to 'divide 5 by 8', and the result of doing the division. Up to now in the book we have used the symbol '÷' to indicate division. From now on, however, we will exploit this interpretation of fraction notation as representing a division. So, instead of writing, say, 9 ÷ 15, we can write $^9/_{15}$ (this is also written, more conveniently, as 9/15). And in doing this we get the answer to the division at the same time (albeit in fraction notation): nine divided by fifteen equals nine fifteenths. Later in this chapter we explain: (a) how we can simplify a fraction like $^9/_{15}$ (to $^3/_5$); and (b) express it in decimal form (as 0.6).

How is a fraction interpreted as a ratio?

One way of comparing two quantities is to subtract one from the other and look at their difference. For example, if infant A weighs 3 kg and infant B weighs 5 kg then we could observe that A is 2 kg lighter than B. But we could also compare them by *dividing* one weight by the other. We would then observe that the weight of A is $^3/_5$ of the weight of B.

This important interpretation of fraction notation uses the idea of division as representing a *ratio*. Sometimes the relationship between A and B is described like this: 'the weights are *in the ratio 3:5*' (3:5 is read as 'three to five'). This means exactly the same as saying that the first weight is three fifths of the second.

EXAMPLE 11.3

A patient has been receiving one 8-mg dose of Drug D each day. Following a review the dosage is reduced to a 5-mg dose each day. Compare the new and original doses by ratio.

The new dose is $^5/_8$ of the original dose. This is using a fraction to represent the ratio.

We can also say that the ratio of the new dose to the original dose is 5:8 (five to eight).

What are equivalent fractions?

Equivalent in mathematics means that two things are in some sense the same. If you were to divide the pizza in Figure 11.1 into 10 equal pieces and took 6 of these, then you would have $^6/_{10}$ of a pizza. This would clearly be the same amount of pizza as the $^3/_5$ shown in Figure 11.1. So we say that $^6/_{10}$ and $^3/_5$ are *equivalent fractions*.

We can easily explain why they are the same: it is because a fifth of a pizza cut in half is the same as two tenths. So the 6 tenths must be the same as 3 fifths. This means that when we change the tenths into fifths, we divide the number of them by 2. This process when applied to a fraction is called *cancelling*. We say that we 'cancel 2'. Effectively this means dividing the top and bottom numbers both by 2. Here are some examples of cancelling 2 to get an equivalent fraction:

Cancelling

A fraction can be made into an equivalent fraction by dividing the top and bottom numbers by the same thing. For example, dividing both by 3:

$$^6/_9 = ^2/_3$$

This is called *cancelling* 3.

$$^6/_8 = ^3/_4 \qquad ^{10}/_{16} = ^5/_8 \qquad ^2/_4 = ^1/_2$$

In each of these examples, the top and bottom numbers in the fraction are both divided by 2. In a similar way, we could divide the fifths in our pizza into 15ths and we would get the same amount of pizza by taking 9 of these. So, $^9/_{15}$ is also equivalent to $^3/_5$. Now we are dividing top and bottom by 3, or cancelling 3. And so it goes on. Any fraction can be made into an equivalent fraction by dividing the top and bottom numbers by the same thing. Here are some examples:

$$^9/_{15} = ^3/_5 \text{ (cancelling 3)} \qquad ^{10}/_{15} = ^2/_3 \text{ (cancelling 5)}$$

$$^6/_{12} = ^1/_2 \text{ (cancelling 6)} \qquad ^{1100}/_{1200} = ^{11}/_{12} \text{ (cancelling 100)}$$

To simplify a fraction by cancelling you look at the *factors* of the numerator and denominator (numbers that divide into them) and identify any factors they have in common. These can then be cancelled. For example, given $^{12}/_{18}$ we might spot that 12 and 18 have 2, 3 and 6 as common factors, so any of these could be cancelled to generate an equivalent fraction:

Simplifying fractions

To get the simplest equivalent fraction divide top and bottom by the *highest common factor.*

$$^{16}/_{24} = ^2/_3 \text{ (cancelling 8)}$$

8 is the highest common factor of 16 and 24.

$$^{12}/_{18} = ^6/_{12} \qquad \text{(cancelling 2)}$$

$$^{12}/_{18} = ^4/_6 \qquad \text{(cancelling 3)}$$

$$^{12}/_{18} = ^2/_3 \qquad \text{(cancelling 6)}$$

Clearly, you get to the simplest equivalent fraction ($^2/_3$) most quickly by cancelling the *highest common factor* (in this case, the 6).

For an example of cancelling, see *Spot the errors* Statement 5 and its correction.

EXAMPLE 11.4

A total dosage of 15 g of Drug E is to be given in 20 equal doses. So each dose will be 15 g divided by 20, which is $^{15}/_{20}$ of a gram. This simplifies to $^3/_4$ of a gram (cancelling 5). In practice this would then be expressed as a decimal, as explained later in this chapter. See check-up question 11.8.

More simplification

Sometimes a simpler equivalent fraction is obtained by multiplying the top and bottom by the same number. For example, multiplying both by 4:

$$^{0.25}/_2 = ^1/_8$$

Just as you can get an equivalent fraction by dividing top and bottom of a fraction by the same number, you can also use the inverse operation: multiply top and bottom by the same number. This is particularly useful when one or more of the numbers involved in the fraction is a decimal. For example, if the fraction $^{2.7}/_3$ turned up in a calculation we could simplify this by multiplying top and bottom by 10, to get $^{27}/_{30}$. We can then cancel 3 to simplify this further as $^9/_{10}$. Look back at our explanation of division involving decimal numbers in Chapter 9 and you will see that we have already made use of this approach for making division of decimals easier (Examples 9.13 and 9.14).

EXAMPLE 11.5

A bandage is 6 m long. If a length of 4.4 m has been used, what fraction of the bandage remains?

The length remaining is 1.6 m, so the fraction remaining is $^{1.6}/_6$ of the roll. Multiply top and bottom by 10 and this fraction simplifies to $^{16}/_{60}$. This can be simplified further by cancelling 4, to give $^4/_{15}$ of the roll.

EXAMPLE 11.6

When Drug E is reconstituted the solution has a concentration of 0.4 mg per ml. The nurse correctly writes down that to provide a dose of 5 mg of Drug E a volume of $^5/_{0.4}$ ml is required. (This kind of calculation is explained in Chapter 12.) The nurse needs to simplify this result.

Multiplying top and bottom of $^5/_{0.4}$ by 10 will get rid of the decimal point. This gives the fraction $^5/_{0.4}$ as being equal to $^{50}/_4$. Cancel 2 and this becomes $^{25}/_2$. The volume is $^{25}/_2$ ml. This result is a 'top-heavy fraction', which could then be expressed as $12^1/_2$ ml, a 'mixed number' (these ideas are explained later in the chapter; see Example 11.9).

What are equivalent ratios?

Since one of the interpretations of fractions is as ratios, it follows that we can generate *equivalent ratios* in the same way: by multiplying or dividing both numbers in the ratio by the same number.

EXAMPLE 11.7

If there are 48 male healthcare workers and 120 female healthcare workers in a hospital department, the ratio of male to female is 48:120. This can be simplified to an equivalent ratio by dividing both numbers by 12, giving a ratio of 4:10, which can be simplified further (by dividing both numbers by 2) to a ratio of 2:5. This means that for every 2 male workers there are 5 female.

EXAMPLE 11.8

A patient has been receiving a 50-microgram dose of Drug F each day. Following a review this is reduced to a 40-microgram dose each day. Compare the doses by ratio.

The ratio of the new dose to the previous dose is 40:50. This can be simplified to a ratio of 4:5 (dividing both numbers by 10).

In a ratio either of the two quantities involved can be written first. So, in Example 11.7 we could turn the statement round and say that the ratio of females to males is 5:2. In Example 11.8 we could say that the ratio of the previous dose to the new dose is 5:4.

How do you express a ratio as 'one to something' or 'something to one'?

A common device is to express a ratio as 'one to something', or 'something to one'. This is often used, for example, in scales on maps. The reader may be familiar with Ordnance Survey maps with a scale such as 1:50 000. This means that 1 cm on the map represents 50 000 cm in reality.

Similarly, we could express the ratio in Example 11.7 as 'one to something'. To do this we divide both numbers in the ratio 2:5 by the first number, 2, to get the ratio 1:2.5. This would then be interpreted something like this: for every one male worker there are 2.5 female. It means that the number of female workers is 2.5 times the number of male workers. Or we could express this ratio as 'something to one', by dividing both numbers by the second number, 5, to get the ratio 0.4:1. This means: there are 0.4 male workers for every one female worker. So, the number of male workers is 0.4 times the number of female workers.

In Chapter 12 we will explain calculations involving *concentrations*. A concentration is an example of a ratio expressed as 'something to one'. For example, if a solution

Equivalent ratios

Simplifying ratios works just the same as simplifying fractions, by dividing (or multiplying) both numbers in the ratio by the same number.

6:10 = 3:5 (dividing both by 2)

1.7:2 = 17:20 (multiplying both by 10)

2.25:25 = 9:100 (multiplying both by 4)

6:9 = 1:1.5 (dividing both by 6)

contains 250 mg of a drug in 100 ml of a solution, then the ratio of milligrams of the drug to millilitres of the solution is 250:100. This is equivalent to 2.5:1. This means that in each 1 millilitre of solution there are 2.5 mg of the drug. This is what we mean when we say that the concentration is 2.5 mg per ml.

Can you have a fraction greater than 1? What are mixed numbers?

Mixed numbers

Some examples

$$^3/_2 = 1^1/_2$$

$$^7/_2 = 3^1/_2$$

$$^7/_4 = 1^3/_4$$

$$^{10}/_3 = 3^1/_3$$

$$^{25}/_4 = 6^1/_4$$

Yes, you can have a fraction greater than 1. These are fractions where the top number is greater than the bottom number. In relation to Figure 11.1, for example, we could imagine 3 pizzas cut into fifths and some particularly greedy person taking 11 slices. It makes sense to describe what they have as $^{11}/_5$ (eleven fifths) of a pizza. We could call this a 'top-heavy' fraction. This is clearly more than 1 pizza. In fact it is equivalent to 2 pizzas and $^1/_5$ of a pizza. This is often written as what is called a *mixed number*, like this: $2^1/_5$ (which is read as 'two and one fifth').

EXAMPLE 11.9

(a) The result of Example 11.6 was $^{25}/_2$ ml (twenty-five halves). Since 24 halves are equivalent to 12 whole units, $^{25}/_2$ can be written as $12^1/_2$ ml.

(b) (Compare Example 11.2) A total dosage of 15 g of Drug G is to be given in 4 equal doses. So each dose will be 15 g divided by 4, which is $^{15}/_4$ (fifteen quarters) of a gram. Now 12 quarters of a unit make 3 whole units ($3 \times 4 = 12$). So 15 quarters is 3 whole units and 3 more quarters. So, written as a mixed number, $^{15}/_4$ of a gram is $3^3/_4$ (three and three quarters) grams.

The results of (a) and (b) would then be written in decimal form: see check-up question 11.8.

Changing fractions to decimals

Make sure you can write down immediately the decimal equivalents of any number of tenths, hundredths and thousandths; and know by heart the decimal equivalents of a half, quarters and fifths (at least).

Which fractions have simple equivalences as decimal numbers?

In healthcare practice most calculations are done with decimal numbers rather than with fractions. Many fractions can be easily converted to decimal numbers mentally – and it is really helpful to have the most common equivalences between fractions and decimal numbers at your fingertips.

To start with we have the tenths. The first place in a decimal number represents tenths: 0.1 is 1 tenth; 0.2 is 2 tenths; 0.3 is 3 tenths and so on. This principle gives us some easy equivalences between fractions and decimal numbers. For example:

$$^1/_{10} = 0.1 \qquad ^3/_{10} = 0.3 \qquad ^7/_{10} = 0.7 \qquad ^9/_{10} = 0.9$$

In the same way, we can change hundredths straight into decimal numbers, for example:

$$^1/_{100} = 0.01 \quad ^7/_{100} = 0.07 \quad ^{19}/_{100} = 0.19 \quad ^{37}/_{100} = 0.37 \quad ^{99}/_{100} = 0.99$$

And thousandths, likewise:

$$^1/_{1000} = 0.001 \; ^7/_{1000} = 0.007 \; ^{23}/_{1000} = 0.023 \; ^{707}/_{1000} = 0.707 \; ^{999}/_{1000} = 0.999$$

More fun is recognizing the decimal equivalents of other fractions. Look out for those where the denominator is a factor of 10, a factor of 100, or a factor of 1000. In particular, you should be able quickly to convert fractions with denominators of 2, 4, 5, 8, 25 and 50 into decimal numbers. This is done by converting the fraction mentally into an equivalent fraction, with 10, 100 or 1000 as the denominator.

Here are some examples, which you should definitely know by heart:

$^1/_2 = ^5/_{10}$ (multiplying top and bottom by 5) so $^1/_2 = 0.5$

$^1/_5 = ^2/_{10}$ (multiplying top and bottom by 2) so $^1/_5 = 0.2$

$^2/_5 = ^4/_{10}$ (multiplying top and bottom by 2) so $^2/_5 = 0.4$

$^3/_5 = ^6/_{10}$ (multiplying top and bottom by 2) so $^3/_5 = 0.6$

$^4/_5 = ^8/_{10}$ (multiplying top and bottom by 2) so $^4/_5 = 0.8$

$^1/_4 = ^{25}/_{100}$ (multiplying top and bottom by 25) so $^1/_4 = 0.25$

$^3/_4 = ^{75}/_{100}$ (multiplying top and bottom by 25) so $^3/_4 = 0.75$

Here are some further examples, which if you do not memorize you should at least be able to deduce quickly:

$^1/_8 = ^{125}/_{1000}$ (multiplying top and bottom by 125) so $^1/_8 = 0.125$

$^1/_{25} = ^4/_{100}$ (multiplying top and bottom by 4) so $^1/_{25} = 0.04$

$^1/_{50} = ^2/_{100}$ (multiplying top and bottom by 2) so $^1/_{50} = 0.02$

Other fractions with these denominators can then be deduced quickly, as shown below. Because $^1/_8 = 0.125$:

$^3/_8$ will be 0.125 multiplied by 3, so $^3/_8 = 0.375$

$^5/_8$ will be 0.125 multiplied by 5, so $^5/_8 = 0.625$

$^7/_8 =$ will be 0.125 multiplied by 7, so $^7/_8 = 0.875$

Because $^1/_{25} = 0.04$:

$^2/_{25}$ will be 0.04 multiplied by 2, so $^2/_{25} = 0.08$

$^{24}/_{25}$ will be 0.04 multiplied by 24, so $^{24}/_{25} = 0.96$

Because $^1/_{50} = 0.02$:

$^3/_{50}$ will be 0.02 multiplied by 3, so $^3/_{50} = 0.06$

$^{49}/_{50}$ will be 0.02 multiplied by 49, so $^{49}/_{50} = 0.98$.

EXAMPLE 11.10

A patient-controlled analgesia infusion contains 16 mg of morphine in 50 ml. The concentration of morphine in the infusion preparation is written down correctly as $^{16}/_{50}$ of a milligram per millilitre (see Chapter 12), which is cancelled down to $^8/_{25}$ mg per ml. Express this as a decimal.

We know that $^1/_{25} = 0.04$, so $^8/_{25}$ will be 0.04 multiplied by 8, which is 0.32. So the concentration of morphine is 0.32 mg per ml.

Alternatively, we could multiply top and bottom of $^{16}/_{50}$ by 2, to get the equivalent fraction $^{32}/_{100}$, which we should know immediately to be equal to 0.32.

EXAMPLE 11.11

(Spot the errors statement 11 corrected)

If $^5/_8$ of a litre of a suspension has been infused then the volume that has been infused is 0.125 litres multiplied by 5 (because $^1/_8 = 0.125$), which equals 0.625 litres (or 625 ml).

What are the decimal equivalents of $^1/_3$ and $^2/_3$?

Above we have listed a number of fractions for which you should expect to remember their decimal equivalents or be able to work them out mentally, without too much difficulty. But clearly none of us can remember the decimal equivalents for all fractions, so we need a method for working them out. This is important because dosages will in practice be expressed in decimal form rather than in fractional notation.

We will start with two familiar fractions, for which you may well already know the decimal equivalents: $^1/_3$ and $^2/_3$ (one third and two thirds). To write $^1/_3$ as a decimal, remember that one of the meanings of $^1/_3$ is '1 divided by 3'. So that is all we have to do!

To convert $1/_3$ to decimal form: divide 1 by 3. We could do this by writing 1 as 1.0000…
and using short division. (See Figure 11.3.)

$$\frac{0.3\ 3\ 3\ …}{3\,\overline{\,1.0^1 0^1 0^1 0\ 0\ …\,}}$$

Figure 11.3   Calculating $1/_3$ as a decimal by short division

As we do this division it becomes clear very soon that the
result is going to be 0.3333333…, with the 3s going on
forever. Each time we divide 10 by 3 we get remainder 1
which gives us 10 in the next column to divide by 3! The
result is called a *recurring decimal* – a decimal number in
which one or more digits repeat themselves forever. This
means that we cannot write down $1/_3$ exactly as a decimal
and will have to round it to an appropriate level of accuracy. For most practical purposes we can take $1/_3$ to be
equal to 0.333 (to 3 significant digits).

   Doubling 0.3333333… we get the value of $2/_3$ to be the
recurring decimal 0.6666666…, which rounds to 0.667 (to
3 significant digits). Notice that if we just double 0.333 we
get 0.666, rather than 0.667: this is the result of a rounding
error. (See Chapter 8.)

How do you convert other fractions into an equivalent decimal?

In general, to change a fraction to a decimal we have
three choices: (a) use decimal equivalences we already
know to work it out mentally; (b) use a written method
to do the division calculation; (c) do the division on a
calculator. Here are some examples to illustrate these
choices:

- Express $0.1/_3$ as a decimal. We can relate this to $1/_3 = 0.333$
  (to 3 significant digits) and do it mentally. Since the 0.1 being
  divided is a tenth of 1, the answer will be a tenth of $1/_3$, which
  gives $0.1/_3 = 0.0333$ (to 3 significant digits).
- Express $2/_9$ as a decimal. We might do this by dividing 2 by
  9, using short division (see Figure 11.3 where this method is
  used for 1 ÷ 3), to get the result 0.222 (to 3 significant digits).
- Express $1.7/_{24}$ as a decimal. Dividing 1.7 by 24 is rather tricky,
  so any sane person would use a calculator: 1.7 ÷ 24 = 0.0708
  (to 3 significant digits).

Thirds as decimals

Results to remember

To three significant digits

$1/_3 = 0.333$

$2/_3 = 0.667$

To change a fraction to a decimal

(1) If you can, relate the fraction to another fraction for
which you already know
the decimal equivalent.

(2) You can always just divide
the numerator by the
denominator. Do this by
mental methods, written
methods, or on a calcula-
tor, as appropriate.

EXAMPLE 11.12

A total volume of 200 ml of a preparation is to be infused over 30 minutes. The infusion rate (see Chapter 12) is correctly calculated as $200/30 = {}^{20}/_3$ ml per minute. Express this as a decimal.

We could do this mentally. We know ${}^2/_3 = 0.667$ (approximately), so we can easily find ${}^{20}/_3$. Because 20 divided by 3 is clearly 10 times greater than 2 divided by 3, the value of ${}^{20}/_3$ has to be 10 times greater than ${}^2/_3$. So ${}^{20}/_3 = 0.667 \times 10 = 6.67$. The infusion rate is 6.67 ml per minute. In practice this may be rounded to 7 ml per minute.

EXAMPLE 11.13

After 5 hours of a 12-hour infusion, ${}^5/_{12}$ of a litre of a preparation has been infused. What is this volume expressed as a decimal? We have to calculate $5 \div 12$. If we are confident with multiples of 12 we could do this by short division. Or, using a calculator, $5 \div 12 = 0.417$ (to 3 significant digits). So the volume that has been infused is 0.417 litres (417 ml).

How do you write mixed numbers in decimal form?

Occasionally we need to write a mixed number as a decimal number. For example, we might have deduced correctly that a dose of a drug should be $12^2/_5$ mg. In practice dosages are expressed in decimal form, so what is $12^2/_5$ written as a decimal? Well, it is only the fractional part (${}^2/_5$) of the mixed number that needs attention. The whole number part, 12, will stay as 12 in front of the decimal point. Since ${}^2/_5 = 0.4$, then we have $12^2/_5$ mg = 12.4 mg.

How do you convert a decimal into a fraction?

To change a decimal to a fraction

Write the decimal number as tenths or hundredths or thousandths, and then simplify as much as possible by cancelling.

Sometimes in the middle of a calculation with decimals it helps to think of a decimal number as a fraction. For example, you might find the calculation 0.125×40 easier to do if you spot that 0.125 is just ${}^1/_8$. (${}^1/_8 \times 40$ is one eighth of 40, which is 5.) It will certainly increase your confidence in calculations if you can move freely between fractions and decimals, in either direction. All the common equivalences that have been memorized can be applied in reverse, of course ($0.5 = {}^1/_2$; $0.75 = {}^3/_4$; $0.4 = {}^2/_5$, $0.375 = {}^3/_8$, and so on).

Otherwise all that is involved in changing a decimal number to a fraction is to express it as so many tenths, or hundredths, or thousandths, and then to simplify it as much as possible by cancelling.

EXAMPLE 11.14

Express in fraction form: (a) 0.7 litres; (b) 0.35 g; (c) 3.125 mg.

(a) A number with only one digit after the decimal point can be written in tenths. So, 0.7 litres = $^7/_{10}$ litres. This cannot be simplified further.

(b) A number with two digits after the decimal point can be written in hundredths. So, 0.35 g = $^{35}/_{100}$ of a gram. Cancelling 5, this simplifies to $^7/_{20}$ of a gram.

(c) Only the bit after the decimal point needs to be changed to a fraction. This is 0.125, which we remember is $^1/_8$. So 3.125 mg = $3^1/_8$ mg.

How do you calculate a fraction of a quantity?

We finally get to the most common calculation involving fractions: finding a fraction of a number or quantity. For example: finding $^2/_3$ of a packet of 24 tablets; $^3/_5$ of 1000 ml; $^5/_8$ of 120 mg.

Finding a fraction of a quantity

To find a fraction $^a/_b$ of a quantity, divide by b and then multiply by a.

We will start with a simple, everyday example, with which you are familiar. What is $^1/_4$ of an hour in minutes? In other words what is $^1/_4$ of 60 minutes? This just means dividing the 60 into 4 equal parts. Hence, $^1/_4$ of 60 = 60 ÷ 4 = 15. So, as we know, a quarter of an hour is 15 minutes.

So, here's the first thing to be absolutely clear about:

$^1/_4$ of a number = the number divided by 4

$^1/_3$ of a number = the number divided by 3

$^1/_5$ of a number = the number divided by 5, and so on.

Hence we have: $^1/_4$ of 60 = 15, $^1/_3$ of 60 = 20; $^1/_5$ of 60 = 12, and so on. So, what is $^3/_4$ of an hour in minutes? Saying this in words tells us what to do: '*three* quarters of 60' is *one* quarter of 60, multiplied by 3, hence 45 minutes.

So, if you want to find $^2/_3$ (two thirds) of a number or quantity, you first find one third (divide by 3) and then multiply by 2. If you want to find $^3/_5$ (three fifths) of something, you first find one fifth (divide by 5) and then multiply by 3.

EXAMPLE 11.15

(a) How many tablets in $^2/_3$ of a packet of 24 tablets?

Divide 24 by 3 to get $^1/_3$ of 24 tablets = 8 tablets.

Then multiply by 2 to get $^2/_3$ of 24 tablets = 16 tablets.

(b) What is $^3/_5$ of 1000 ml?

Divide 1000 by 5 to get $^1/_5$ of 1000 ml = 200 ml.

Then multiply by 3 to get $^3/_5$ of 1000 ml = 600 ml.

(c) Find $^5/_8$ of 120 mg.

Divide 120 by 8 to get $^1/_8$ of 120 mg = 15 mg.

Then multiply by 5 to get $^5/_8$ of 120 mg = 75 mg.

If the calculations get too tricky to handle mentally, use a calculator, but follow the same process.

EXAMPLE 11.16

After 21 hours, $^7/_8$ of a 24-hour infusion of 1500 ml has been delivered (because $^{21}/_{24} = ^7/_8$). What volume has been delivered?

We need to find $^7/_8$ of 1500, so we must divide by 8 and multiply by 7.

On a calculator, enter 1500 ÷ 8 × 7, getting the result 1312.5. So the volume delivered so far is about 1310 ml (to 3 significant digits).

11.1 So far, 12 boxes of Ibuprofen from a pharmacy's stock of 20 boxes have been used.

  (a) What fraction of the stock has been used? Give the answer in its simplest form.

  (b) What fraction of the stock remains?

11.2 If a volume of 3 litres of water is shared equally between 18 beakers, what fraction of a litre would there be in each beaker? Give the answer in its simplest form.

11.3   In an imaginary world a practice nurse is given a pay rise of £50 a month while the secretary is given a rise of £35 a month.

(a) Complete this sentence with a fraction in its simplest form: the secretary's rise is ☐ of the nurse's rise.

(b) What is the ratio of the secretary's rise to the nurse's rise?

11.4   Write in the boxes the numbers required to make all the ratios equivalent to the ratio of 6 to 9.

$6:9 = 2:☐ = ☐:27 = 600:☐ = 1:☐$

11.5   In Example 11.8 earlier in the chapter, the ratio of the original dose to the new dose is 5:4. Express this ratio:

(a) as 'one to something'

(b) as 'something to one'

11.6   An infusion rate of 22.5 ml per hour is equal to $^{22.5}/_{60}$ ml per minute.

(a) Simplify this fraction.

(b) Write the rate in ml per minute in decimal form.

11.7   If 25 mg of Drug H is to be given in 4 equal doses, each dose is $^{25}/_4$ mg.

(a) Write this top-heavy fraction as a mixed number.

(b) Then write the dose in decimal form.

11.8   Give the results in Examples 11.2, 11.4, and 11.9(a) and (b), from earlier in this chapter, in decimal form.

11.9   Change the following to decimal equivalences:

(a) $^1/_2$ of a degree Celsius   (b) $^1/_4$ of a litre

(c) $^9/_{10}$ of a centimetre   (d) $^7/_{100}$ of a metre

(e) $^7/_8$ of a gram   (f) $^2/_5$ of a litre

(g) $^9/_{25}$ of a milligram   (h) $^3/_{50}$ of a kilogram

(i) $2^1/_4$ millilitres   (j) $^{105}/_{60}$ hours

11.10   Express $^{13}/_3$ as a mixed number and then convert it to decimal form (to 3 significant digits).

11.11   Express the fractions $^1/_6, ^2/_6, ^3/_6, ^4/_6$ and $^5/_6$ as decimals (to no more than 3 significant digits).

(Continued)

(Continued)

11.12   A patient-controlled analgesia infusion contains 2.5 mg of morphine in 30 ml. The concentration of morphine in the infusion preparation is calculated as $^{2.5}/_{30}$ of a milligram per millilitre. Convert this to an equivalent fraction with 5 as the numerator and then use one of your answers from the previous check-up question (11.11) to write this result as a decimal.

11.13   A total of 50 mg of Drug J is to be taken in 6 equal doses. Each dose will be $^{50}/_{6}$ mg. Express this dose in decimal form (to 3 significant digits).

11.14   Use a calculator to express the following quantities in decimal form (without changing the units of measurement) to three significant digits:

(a) $^{5}/_{24}$ of a litre   (b) $^{17}/_{60}$ of an hour

(c) $^{3}/_{125}$ of a kilogram

11.15   A consultant calculates that a patient with a skin condition should receive light treatment for 2.4 hours.

(a) This is 2 hours and what fraction of an hour?

(b) This is 2 hours and how many minutes?

11.16   Express as fractions, in their simplest forms:

(a) 0.9 litres   (b) 0.08 g

(c) 0.125 m   (d) 3.25 mg

11.17   (a) An infusion is to be delivered over 12 hours. After $7^{1}/_{2}$ hours what fraction of the total volume has been delivered? Give the answer as a fraction in its simplest form.

(b) If the infusion is 1000 ml in total, what volume has been delivered in the $7^{1}/_{2}$ hours?

11.18   (a) How many tablets in $^{3}/_{5}$ of a packet of 40 tablets?

(b) What is $^{7}/_{8}$ of 600 ml?

(c) Find $^{5}/_{6}$ of 120 mg.

PROPORTIONALITY AND 'PER'

12

OBJECTIVES

In a practical healthcare context the practitioner should be able to:

- recognize the two variables in a proportional relationship and the given values of these
- solve simple problems of proportion
- interpret the word 'per' in the many situations in which it arises
- do calculations involving dosage per kilogram of body weight
- do calculations involving dosage per square metre of body surface area
- do calculations involving drug concentration (per millilitre, per litre)
- do calculations involving infusion rates (per hour, per minute)
- calculate drop rates for an infusion

The subject matter of this chapter relates to a large number of the dosage and infusion calculations involved in healthcare practice. It is absolutely crucial that practitioners can handle proportional relationships with confidence and accuracy. In discussing this topic we aim to encourage you to understand the principles of proportionality and to exploit any obvious relationships between the numbers involved, rather than relying only on memorizing and applying rules for different kinds of drug and infusion calculations.

SPOT THE ERRORS

Identify any obvious errors in the calculations in the following eight statements.

1   Drug A is supplied as an oral solution containing 100 mg in 5 ml and a patient has been prescribed 250 mg, so the volume to be given to the patient is 12.5 ml.

2   If 5 ml of a preparation delivers 200 mg of Drug B then to deliver 120 mg of Drug B the volume needed is 2.2 ml.

3   If a child is prescribed 7.5 mg of metronidazole per kg of body weight every 8 hours and the child weighs 28 kg then the 8-hourly dose required is $7.5 \times 28 = 210$ mg.

4   A vial of Drug C contains a total volume of 50 ml with a concentration of 5 mg per ml. For a patient requiring 200 mg of Drug C intravenously as a slow infusion the volume to be administered is $200/50 \times 5 = 20$ ml.

5   Dobutamine with a concentration of 12.5 mg per ml is available as stock in an ampoule containing 20 ml, so each ampoule contains a dosage of $12.5 \times 20 = 250$ mg of dobutamine.

6   If the recommended weekly injection of doxorubicin for a child with leukaemia is a dosage of 30 mg per square metre of body surface area, then the recommended dosage for a child with body surface area of 0.42 square metres is $30 \div 0.42 = 71.4$ mg (rounded to one decimal place).

7   If 500 ml of dextrose 5% is to be infused over 4 hours, then the infusion rate is 125 ml per hour.

8   The rate for a continuous intravenous infusion of heparin is given as 18 units per kg per hour; for a patient weighing 75 kg this will be $75 \times 18 = 1350$ units per hour.

Are the errors you have spotted potentially serious in medical health practice?

(errors identified on page 148)

What is a proportional relationship?

We introduced the idea of proportionality towards the end of Chapter 10, in the context of converting measurements between metric and imperial units. All the examples we use here in Chapter 12 will have the same mathematical structure as the examples given there.

First, there will be two *variables*. A variable is a quantity that theoretically can take any value in a given range. Here are some examples of variables that we will use in this chapter:

- the weight of an adult patient measured in kilograms
- the body surface area of a child patient measured in square metres (m^2)
- the dosage (weight) of a particular drug measured in mg to be given to a patient
- the volume in ml of a preparation delivered to a patient by infusion
- the time required for an infusion, measured in hours.

So, proportionality is a relationship between two variables like these. The relationship is such that when the value of one variable changes then so does the value of the other variable change, but always in the same ratio. This means that the relationship between the variables can be defined by multiplication and division, as we illustrate in the following example.

EXAMPLE 12.1

An infusion is set up to deliver 750 ml in 6 hours.

The two variables that describe the progress of the infusion are:

(a) the volume in ml that has been infused,

(b) the time in hours that the infusion has been running.

What volume has been infused in 2 hours? Answer: 250 ml.

The time of 6 hours is 3 times as long as the given time of 2 hours.

So the volume infused in 6 hours will be 3 times the volume infused in 2 hours.

And the volume infused in 2 hours will be the volume infused in 6 hours divided by 3.

ERRORS IDENTIFIED

The obvious errors are Statements 2, 4 and 6.

Statement 2

The volume required is 3 ml. This statement has the typical structure of a question based on a proportional relationship between two variables: the volume of the preparation in ml and the amount of Drug B in mg. We explain how to work with this kind of proportional relationship in this chapter. (See Example 12.2(b).)

Statement 4

The volume required is 40 ml. This is a typical question about concentration and volume. The key information given is the concentration (5 mg per ml) and the dosage in mg of Drug C required (200 mg). The volume required is 200/5 = 40 ml. (See Example 12.5(b).) The additional information given (that the vial contains 50 ml) is not required in this calculation. After the 40-ml volume required has been calculated the information that the vial contains 50 ml becomes useful because we then know that one vial will be sufficient.

Statement 6

The wrong calculation has been done, resulting in a serious overdose. The calculation required to find the dosage is 30 × 0.42 which gives a dosage of 12.6 mg. (See Example 12.7(b).)

All the statements here are using the principles of a proportional relationship between two variables. Many calculations of drug dosage and infusion rate calculations require confidence and accuracy in the application of this kind of mathematical reasoning. Errors such as those in Statements 2, 4 and 6 are potentially very serious in relation to the well-being of the patient. Statements 2 and 4 result in the patients receiving insufficient dosages, whereas Statement 6 would lead to a serious overdose which could be potentially life-threatening. Statement 2 is an actual answer given on a test paper by a trainee nurse, who clearly has very little clue about how to deal with proportional relationships. Our intention is that by studying this chapter carefully you will ensure that you are not equally mystified by the principles of proportionality.

(now continue reading from page 147)

Figure 12.1 shows the four numbers involved in Example 12.1, arranged in a two-by-two array of four boxes: two values of the volume (in ml) and the corresponding two values of the time (in hours). Looking at the numbers in the columns, we see that the ratio 250:750 is the same as the ratio 2:6 (they both simplify to 1:3). Similarly, looking at the numbers in the rows we see that the ratio 250:2 is the same as the ratio 750:6.

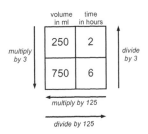

Figure 12.1   The relationships between the variables in Example 12.1

This simple arrangement of the data helps us to identify the satisfying pattern of relationships between the values of the variables. First, looking at the columns, you can get from the values on the column on the right to the corresponding values on the left by multiplying by 125. Or you can go in the reverse direction by dividing by 125. You can also do the same thing with the rows: multiplying the values in the top row by 3 to get those in the bottom row; or dividing the values in the bottom row by 3 to get those in the top row. This pattern of multiplication and division is the key to understanding and therefore to solving problems of proportionality. (Note: as we stated in Chapter 10, what we are describing here is strictly called *direct* proportionality.)

How do you solve problems of proportionality?

Look for the obvious

Many problems of proportion can be solved informally by exploiting the most obvious multiplication and division relationships between the given values of the variables.

Many problems of proportionality can be solved informally by using simple multiplications and divisions. The two-by-two array will help us to organize the data in a way that helps us to spot and exploit the simplest relationships between the values involved.

A problem of proportionality will always include two values of each of the two variables. The four numbers involved can be arranged in a two-by-two array, as shown in Figure 12.1. Of these four numbers, three will be known or given and the fourth will have to be calculated. To find the missing number you can use any multiplications or divisions like those shown in Figure 12.1. Which you choose to use may depend on the numbers involved. For example, if you see, say, 25 and 100 in the same row, you should be expecting to multiply or divide by 4 to solve the problem (because 100 is 4 times 25). Or, if you see 120 and 6 in the same column, you will be expecting to multiply or divide by 20 (because 120 is 20 times 6).

EXAMPLE 12.2

(a) Drug D is available as a suspension containing 250 mg in 5 ml. What volume is required to administer a dose of 1000 mg (1 g)?

The two variables are the dose of Drug D in milligrams and the volume of the suspension in ml. Figure 12.2(a) shows the three given values arranged in a two-by-two array. The question mark is what is to be calculated: the volume in ml corresponding to the dose of 1000 mg. The easiest way to find this value is to notice that the 250 is multiplied by 4 to get the 1000, so the 5 also gets multiplied by 4, to give the result 20 ml.

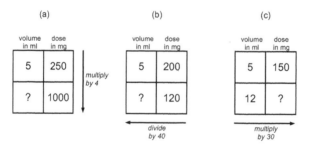

Figure 12.2   Three values are known, one is to be found (Example 12.2)

(b) (Spot the errors Statement 2 corrected) If 5 ml of a preparation delivers 200 mg of Drug E then what volume is needed to deliver 120 mg?

The two variables are the dose of Drug E in milligrams and the volume of the oral suspension in ml. Figure 12.2(b) shows the three given values arranged in a two-by-two array. The question mark is what is to be calculated: the volume in ml corresponding to the dose of 120 mg. Looking at the numbers here we might spot that to get from the 200 to the 5 we divide by 40. So the 120 must also be divided by 40 (120/40 = 3); the volume required = 3 ml.

(c) An oral solution contains 150 mg of Drug F in 5 ml. A patient is given 12 ml of this oral solution. What dose of Drug F in milligrams does this contain?

Once again the two variables are the dose in mg and the volume in ml. Figure 12.2 (c) shows the three given values, with the question mark indicating the value to be found. Here we might spot that you get from the 5 to the 150 by multiplying by 30. So the 12 must also be multiplied by 30 ($30 \times 12 = 360$); the dose of Drug F being given is 360 mg.

Another way of explaining what is going on here is to think in terms of finding 'equivalent ratios' (see Chapter 11).

In Example 12.2(a) we are given the ratio of millilitres to milligrams as 5:250. Multiplying both numbers by 4 gives us the equivalent ratio, 20:1000. Hence 20 ml is required to provide 1000 mg.

In Example 12.2(b) we are given the ratio of millilitres to milligrams as 5:200. First simplify this to 1:40 (dividing both numbers by 5). Then multiplying both numbers by 3 gives us the equivalent ratio, 3:120. Hence 3 ml is required to provide 120 mg.

In Example 12.2(c) we are given the ratio of millilitres to milligrams as 5:150. First simplify this to 1:30 (dividing both numbers by 5). Then multiplying both numbers by 12 gives us the equivalent ratio, 12:360. Hence 12 ml provides 360 mg.

But sometimes there will not be an easy, obvious relationship that you can spot immediately between the numbers involved. When this is the case you may need to do some trickier calculations to identify what you multiply by to get from one column (or row) to the other, maybe using a calculator to help you.

EXAMPLE 12.3

A child requires 250 mg of paracetamol as a single dose. Paracetamol is available as a suspension containing 120 mg in 5 ml. What volume do we need to give to the child? Figure 12.3 shows the three given values involved here and the one to be found.

We may be able to spot that to get from the 5 to the 120 we have to multiply by 24. If we do not spot it, then we could get this factor of 24 by dividing 120 by 5, using whatever method we are comfortable with. Once we have the 24 we can reason that to get from the 250 to the question mark we have to divide by 24. The calculation 250/24 is not especially easy by mental methods and a calculator may be the best option to get the result ($250/24 = 10.4$ to one decimal place). The volume of the suspension required is 10.4 ml.

volume in ml	dose in mg
5	120
?	250

← divide
by 24

Figure 12.3 Finding the volume required in Example 12.3

What about calculations using 'per kilogram of body weight'?

The pervasive 'per'

Notice how often you use the important little word 'per' to relate variables:

- miles per hour
- cost per 100 g
- calories per 100 g
- beats per minute
- payment per hour
- cost per person

Use your familiarity with these everyday uses to help you understand the use of 'per' in a healthcare context.

The little word *per* is one of the most important and pervasive words in mathematics. We have already used it dozens of times in this book – because it is very difficult to do much application of mathematics without it, particularly in the context of healthcare practice. We are all familiar with the use of the word 'per' in such everyday contexts as speed (miles per hour) and rates of pay (so much per hour), and prices of goods (for example, potatoes costing so much per kilogram). The word 'per' means: 'for each'; or 'for every one'. So to say you are driving at a constant speed of 40 miles per hour means that at this speed you would travel 40 miles in each hour. Whenever we see the word 'per' we should recognize that we are entering the territory of a proportional relationship. In the case of a vehicle travelling at a constant speed of 40 miles per hour, for example, the two variables are the distance travelled in miles and the time taken in hours, and these two variables are proportional: the distance in miles is the time in hours multiplied by 40.

In a healthcare context a familiar occurrence of the word 'per' is in measuring pulse rate. A patient's at-rest pulse rate may be recorded, for example, as 84 beats per minute. The two variables here are the number of beats and the time in minutes. To say '84 beats per minute' means simply that in 1 minute the number of beats is 84. In other lengths of time, if the pulse continues at this rate, the number of beats will be proportional to the time. So, we would expect, for example, 168 beats in 2 minutes; or 42 beats in $\frac{1}{2}$ a minute (30 seconds); or 21 beats in $\frac{1}{4}$ of a minute (15 seconds); or 28 beats in $\frac{1}{3}$ of a minute (20 seconds); and so on.

Per kilogram of body weight

Multiplying the dose per kg by the patient's weight in kilograms will give the dose for that patient.

An important example in healthcare practice – to which we have already referred in a number of examples in earlier chapters – is drug dosage given as so many grams or milligrams 'per kilogram of body weight'.

EXAMPLE 12.4

(a) The recommended total daily dose of Drug G is 40 mg per kg of body weight. What total daily dose is recommended for an adult who weighs 75kg?

If the recommended dose is 40 mg 'for each' kilogram of body weight, then for 75 kg the calculation required is just 40×75 (which equals 3000). So the dose is 3000 mg (= 3 g).

(b) Drug H is given to a child at a dose of 20 mg per kg four times daily. What is the dose to be given four times a day to a child weighing 14 kg?

The dose is just 20 mg × 14 = 280 mg of Drug H.

To emphasize the proportionality here, notice that in Example 12.4(a) the '40 mg per kg' could be interpreted as '40 mg for each 1 kg'. This is saying (theoretically) that someone with a body weight of 1 kg gets a dose of 40 mg. We have to use this to find the dose for a body weight of 75 kg. So the questions in Example 12.4 could be represented by Figure 12.4(a) and (b). Of course we would not expect you to have to use these diagrams for deciding what calculation is required in examples as straightforward as these. But there are similar situations, such as those involving concentrations of solutions, where sometimes practitioners get muddled about whether to multiply or divide.

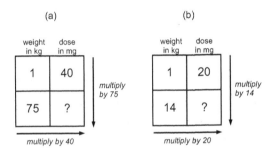

Figure 12.4 Questions involving 'per kilogram' represented in two-by-two arrays

What kinds of dosage calculations involve concentrations?

The concentration of a drug in a solution (or suspension) is the amount of the drug (by weight) in 1 unit of volume of the solution (or suspension). The amount of the drug might be measured in grams, milligrams or micrograms; the unit of volume might be 1 litre or 1 millilitre. So concentrations might be measured in 'mg per ml', or 'g per litre', and so on.

If you know what dosage of a drug (measured, say, in mg) is contained in a certain volume of a solution or suspension (measured, say, in ml), then the concentration (mg per ml) is found just by dividing the dosage by the volume. This is just like calculating your average speed in miles per hour by dividing the number of miles you have travelled by the number of hours it has taken you.

In Example 12.2(a) we were told that Drug D is available as a suspension containing 250 mg in 5 ml. How would we use this information to find the concentration in

> ### Concentration
>
> To calculate a concentration in mg per ml, divide the given dosage (in mg) by the given volume (in ml).
> For example, if a dosage of 75 mg is contained in a volume of 10 ml, the concentration is 75/10 = 7.5 mg per ml.

Symbol for 'per'

Because of the link with division 'per' is often represented by the symbol '/'.
For example a concentration of 7.5 mg per ml may be written 7.5 mg/ml.

mg per ml? This requires finding what dose of Drug D (in mg) is contained in 1 ml of the suspension. If there are 250 mg in 5 ml, it is clear that there are 50 mg in 1 ml. We simply divide the 250 mg by 5, as though we are sharing it equally between the 5 millilitres. So the concentration is 50 mg per ml (this is often written as 50 mg/ml).

Similarly, in Example 12.2(c) we were told that 150 mg of Drug F is contained in 5 ml of an oral solution. So the concentration is 150/5 = 30 mg per ml (or 30 mg/ml).

Usually you will be given the concentration and have to calculate the volume required to deliver a particular dose, as in Example 12.5(a) and (b), below. Example 12.5(c) involves using the concentration to find the dosage contained within a particular volume.

EXAMPLE 12.5

(a) A pregnant woman is prescribed 450 mg of iron dextran by intravenous infusion; this is available as stock in a solution with a concentration of 50 mg per ml. What volume of the solution does the woman require?

The concentration of 50 mg per ml means: '50 mg of iron dextran is contained in 1 ml of the solution'. These two values (50 and 1) are entered into the table in Figure 12.5(a), together with the third value given, the prescribed dose of 450 mg. We have to find the number of millilitres in the remaining box.

To get from the 50 in the milligram column to the 1 in the millilitre column we have to divide by 50 (that is, we divide by the concentration). So, the 450 is divided by 50 (450/50 = 9), giving the required volume of 9 ml.

(Note, you could also do this by spotting that 50 is multiplied by 9 to give 450, and then multiplying the 1 by 9.)

(b) (Spot the errors Statement 4 corrected) Drug C is available as a solution with a concentration of 5 mg per ml. For a patient requiring 200 mg of Drug C intravenously as a slow infusion what is the volume to be administered?

The concentration of 5 mg per ml gives us the two values in the top row of Figure 12.5(b) as 5 and 1. The required dose of 200 mg is entered in the second row. The question mark is the volume required to deliver a dose of 200 mg that we have to calculate.

To get from the column on the left to the one on the right we spot that we have to divide by 5 (which is, of course, the concentration). Dividing the 200 by 5 (200/5 = 40) gives us the required volume as 40 ml.

(Note, you could also do this by spotting that 5 is multiplied by 40 to give 200, and then multiplying the 1 by 40.)

(c) A pregnant woman is given 7.5 ml of a solution of iron dextran by intravenous infusion; the concentration of the solution is 50 mg per ml. What dosage of iron dextran has she received?

The data here is set up in Figure 12.5(c). The concentration of 50 mg per ml gives us 50 and 1 in the top row of the array. The given volume of 7.5 ml is entered in the second row. We have to find the dose in mg corresponding to this.

We now need to work from the column on the right to the column on the left. This involves multiplication by 50 (because you multiply 1 by 50 to get 50). So we have to multiply the 7.5 ml by 50 (that is, multiply by the concentration) to get the corresponding dosage: $7.5 \times 50 = 375$ ml.

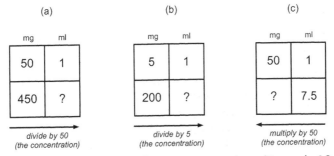

Figure 12.5 Calculations involving concentrations (Example 12.5)

Example 12.5 illustrates the two basic kinds of problems involving concentrations:

- given the concentration and a prescribed dose, find the volume required by *dividing* the dose by the concentration;
- given the concentration and a given volume find the dosage by *multiplying* the volume by the concentration.

Example 12.6 below describes a situation that includes both these procedures.

Calculations using concentration

- volume = dose divided by concentration
- dose = volume multiplied by concentration

EXAMPLE 12.6

Following a normal delivery a neonate requires 1 mg of phytomenadione (vitamin K_1) by intramuscular injection. Phytomenadione with a concentration of 10 mg/ml is available as stock in an ampoule containing 0.2 ml.

(Continued)

(Continued)

(a) Given the volume of 0.2 ml and the concentration of 10 mg/ml we can calculate the dosage of phytomenadione contained in an ampoule to be $0.2 \times 10 = 2$ mg.

(b) Given the dose prescribed of 1 mg and the concentration of 10 mg/ml we can calculate the volume of phytomenadione to be administered to the neonate to be $1/10 = 0.1$ ml.

How do you find a dosage based on body surface area?

First, we will offer a few words of explanation about surface area. The basic idea of area is that it is a measure of the amount of two-dimensional space contained within a boundary. So imagine a field surrounded by a fence; the area is the amount of two-dimensional space bounded by the fence. Area is measured in square units, such as square centimetres or square metres. A square centimetre is the area of a square with side 1 cm. A square metre is the area of a square with side 1 m. Derek's desktop is 2 metres long and 1 metre wide, so it has an area of 2 square metres. This is often written 2 m², with the abbreviation m² standing for 'square metres'. It is not a good idea to read this as 'two metres squared' because this can be confused with the area of a square with side 2 metres, which is actually 4 square metres!

Per square metre of BSA

Multiplying the *dose per m²* by the patient's BSA in square metres will give the dose for that patient.

Area is fairly easy to envisage when applied to two-dimensional (flat) surfaces. But it can also be applied to the surface of a three-dimensional object. For example, the surface area of a full-size football is about 0.15 square metres. This means that if you could peel off the outer surface and somehow spread it flat on a table, then the area of the table covered would be 0.15 m² ($^3/_{20}$ of a square metre). In a similar way we can talk about the surface area of a human body. We are now contemplating the unpleasant image of skinning a human being and spreading the skin out on a table to measure the area it covers! Fortunately, we do not actually have to do this, because there is a formula for estimating the body surface area (BSA), which we will discuss in Chapter 14.

The dosage of some drugs is based on the individual's BSA. In fact the dosage is proportional to the BSA and the drug may therefore be prescribed on the basis of so many milligrams (or grams) per square metre. A prescription that uses 'per square metre' or 'per m²' should be understood to mean 'per square metre of body surface area'.

EXAMPLE 12.7

(a) A cytotoxic medication is prescribed for adults at a dose of 120 mg per square metre as a single dose once every 6 weeks. What dose would be given every 6 weeks to an adult with a BSA of 2.2 m²?

The dose required is 120 mg for each square metre, so for a BSA of 2.2 m^2 we multiply the 120 mg by 2.2, giving the dose as 264 mg.

(b) (Spot the errors Statement 6 corrected) If the recommended weekly injection of doxorubicin for a child with leukaemia is a dosage of 30 mg/m^2, then the recommended dosage for a child with BSA of 0.42 m^2 is 30 × 0.42 = 12.6 mg.

How do you calculate an infusion rate?

Patients who are unable to take or tolerate adequate oral fluids to maintain their fluid and electrolyte requirements, whatever the underlying cause, may require replacement fluids. Replacement fluid is frequently delivered by the intravenous route, because this enables accurate delivery and monitoring. The amount of fluid prescribed for an individual patient is dependent upon a number of factors and will be calculated by the prescrib-

Infusion rate

The infusion rate is the total volume to be infused divided by the time in which the infusion should be completed.

ing clinician following an appropriate assessment. Once the type and volume of fluid have been prescribed along with the time that it is to be infused, a calculation is required to work out the rate at which it is to be infused. We have already used a number of examples of calculations involving infusion rates throughout this book to illustrate various aspects of mathematics. Now we give them the chance to take centre stage.

Infusion rates provide some of the most frequent and important examples in healthcare practice that use our little friend 'per'. This is because the volume being infused is proportional to the time. So, for example, an infusion rate will often be expressed as *millilitres per hour*. The mathematics involved follows the pattern established in this chapter: the rate measured in millilitres per hour (ml/h) is calculated by *dividing* the volume to be infused by the number of hours. Note that the recognized abbreviation for 'hour' is 'h'.

EXAMPLE 12.8

(a) A total volume of 1000 ml of dextrose 5% (see Chapter 13) is to be infused over 8 hours. The infusion rate is the number of millilitres to be infused each hour. To find this we divide 1000 ml by 8 (1000/8 = 125) to determine that the required infusion rate is 125 ml per hour (which might also be written as 125 ml/h).

(b) 1 litre of sodium chloride 0.9% (see Chapter 13) is to be infused over 6 hours. The infusion rate is found by dividing the total volume (1 litre) by 6.

(Continued)

(Continued)

It makes sense to change the volume to 1000 ml before doing the division by 6 (1000/6 = 166.66667). Hence the infusion rate to be set is 167 ml/h (to the nearest millilitre).

Common infusion rates

It is useful to have an idea of the correct rate at which an infusion is to be delivered so that an input error can be identified before the infusion is started. Memorize some common infusion rates. For example: 1000 ml over 8 hours is 125 ml/h. (See check-up question 12.12 at the end of the chapter.)

Rounding the result in Example 12.8(b) to the nearest millilitre would normally be required in practice. It would be very difficult to set a delivery rate for an intravenous infusion with any greater accuracy than to the nearest millilitre. In practice, the delivery of an intravenous infusion to an adult a few minutes early or late will not be of clinical significance. Intravenous infusions can be temperamental and flow rates can be influenced by a number of factors, including the position of the cannula, the patient's movement and the position of the patient's limb. It is essential therefore that the infusion and the patient should be monitored regularly to ensure that the infusion is progressing at the correct rate.

The safest and most reliable way of accurately delivering a large volume of fluid by intravenous infusion is by the use of a volumetric infusion pump. When infusing intravenous fluids to children an infusion pump would always be used, to ensure the higher level of accuracy required. To deliver the fluid at the appropriate rate some basic information is entered into the pump, including the volume to be infused and the time over which the infusion is to be delivered. Once programmed correctly and started the infusion pump will deliver the infusion fluid at a set rate and complete the infusion on time.

Sometimes it is necessary to convert an infusion rate between 'per hour' and 'per minute', as in the following example where the infusion time is only 20 minutes.

EXAMPLE 12.9

A 10-year-old child is to receive an infusion of 45 ml of a metronidazole preparation, to be administered over 20 minutes. At what rate in ml/h should the infusion pump be set?

The infusion rate is again found by dividing the volume by the time, giving 45/20 ml per minute, which is 2.25 ml/min. To convert this to ml per hour, we need to multiply by 60, because there are 60 minutes in an hour, giving 2.25 × 60 = 135 ml/h.

The conversion in Example 12.9 can be done more easily. Because 20 minutes is $\frac{1}{3}$ of an hour the volume delivered in 1 hour will be 3 times the volume delivered in 20 minutes. So the conversion can be done by multiplying 45 by 3 ($45 \times 3 = 135$), giving the infusion rate as 135 ml/h. Because the volume delivered in an hour is proportional to the number of minutes, the data can be set up as shown in Figure 12.6.

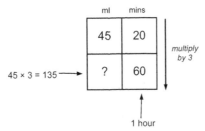

Figure 12.6 Finding the volume delivered in 1 hour (Example 12.9)

In Example 12.10 below the chemical to be administered is provided in solution form in an ampoule. The concentration of this solution is used to calculate the volume (in ml) required to provide a particular dose (in mg). This amount of the solution is then added to a given volume of sodium chloride 0.9% in order to be infused.

EXAMPLE 12.10

A pregnant woman is anaemic and unable to tolerate oral iron preparations; she has been prescribed 1 g (1000 mg) of iron dextran by intravenous infusion. The iron dextran is available as stock in 10-ml ampoules containing 50 mg/ml. This is to be added to 500 ml of sodium chloride 0.9% and infused over 6 hours.

(a) The volume of iron dextran with a concentration of 50 mg/ml required to provide the dose of 1000 mg is 1000/50 = 20 ml. (We note that this volume is provided by 2 complete ampoules.)

(b) When this volume is added to the 500 ml of sodium chloride, the total volume of fluid is 520 ml.

(c) The infusion rate to administer the iron dextran and sodium chloride preparation over 6 hours is 520/6 = 87 ml/h (rounded to the nearest millilitre).

How do you calculate a drop rate?

A standard intravenous giving set delivers:

- 1 ml of clear fluid (such as dextrose 5%, sodium chloride 0.9%, or Hartmann's solution) in 20 drops
- 1 ml of blood in 15 drops.

Standard giving set

- 20 drops per ml of clear fluid

- 15 drops per ml of blood

To work out the drop rate required to deliver accurately an intravenous infusion within the correct time, the volume to be delivered has to be converted into the corresponding number of drops. A drop rate is specified in *drops per minute*, so the calculation requires division of the number of drops by the number of minutes prescribed for the infusion.

EXAMPLE 12.11

Find the drop rate for one litre (1000 ml) of dextrose 5% to be infused over 6 hours, using a standard giving set.

The set delivers 20 drops per ml. So 1000 ml will be delivered in 1000 × 20 = 20 000 drops. The time in hours over which the infusion is to be delivered is converted to minutes: 6 hours x 60 = 360 minutes.

The drop rate is then calculated by dividing the total number of drops by the number of minutes over which the infusion is to be delivered: 20 000/360 = 55.55555 drops per minute, which is 56 drops per minute when rounded to the nearest whole number.

Alternative method: calculate the infusion rate in ml/min (1000/360 = 2.8 ml/h to one decimal place). Since each millilitre is equivalent to 20 drops the number of drops per minute will be 20 times this: 2.8 × 20 = 56 drops/min.

EXAMPLE 12.12

One unit of blood is to be infused over 4 hours; the unit contains 500 ml of blood. Using a standard giving set, what is the correct number of drops per minute required to ensure that the blood runs through on time?

For a blood transfusion the standard giving set delivers 15 drops in 1 millilitre of blood. So for 500 ml, the total number of drops to be delivered is 500 × 15 = 7500 drops.

The time specified for the infusion is 4 hours, which equals 240 minutes.

The drop rate is 7500/240 = 31.25 drops per minute.

This result is rounded to the nearest whole number (31). So the blood would be infused at 31 drops per minute.

Once the rate at which the infusion is to be delivered has been calculated the drops can be counted as they pass through the giving set to ensure that the drop rate is accurate. The rate can be checked and then, if necessary, adjusted by using the roller clamp on the infusion tubing. Once the rate is set the infusion should be checked at regular intervals to ensure that the rate remains correct.

Drop rate

To find the drop rate (drops/min) find the number of drops to be delivered and divide this by the total number of minutes available.

EXAMPLE 12.13

An infusion rate of 56 drops per minute is required. This rate is checked by counting the number of drops over 30 seconds, using a watch with a seconds-hand. Since 30 seconds is half a minute, the number of drops expected in this time is 28. This is equivalent to 14 drops over 15 seconds.

To underline the importance of the mathematical processes in this chapter we have included many more examples for practice in the check-up section that follows. Many healthcare situations require a sequence of calculations, sometimes using more than one of the ideas in this chapter. Examples like this will be given and explained in detail in Chapter 15.

12.1   First, here is an everyday example for practice in using the principles of proportionality. A recipe for a dessert for 4 people requires 360 g of ricotta cheese. This information is entered in the two-by-two arrays in Figure 12.7. Complete these arrays to answer these questions.

(a) What weight of ricotta cheese would be required if this recipe were adapted for 12 people?

(b) What weight of ricotta cheese would be required if this recipe were adapted for 7 people?

(c) For how many people could this recipe be adapted if 550 g of ricotta cheese is available?

HAVE A CHECK-UP

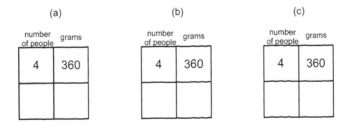

Figure 12.7   Arrays for recipe calculations in check-up question 12.1

(Continued)

(Continued)

12.2   Here are some familiar, everyday examples of calculations using 'per', to reinforce the principles outlined in this chapter.

(a) Potatoes cost £1.50 per kg; what is the cost of 4.5 kg?

(b) A 7-m length of curtain material costs £56; what is the cost per metre?

(c) A car travels at an average speed of 45 miles per hour over a distance of 15
miles; how long does this take?

12.3   (a) A neonate's pulse rate is recorded as 132 beats per minute. At this rate, how
many beats would there be in 15 seconds?

(b) An adult athlete's pulse beats 12 times over 15 seconds. What is the pulse
rate in beats per minute?

12.4   (a) A patient is prescribed 1.5 g (1500 mg) of Drug J as an intravenous injection.
Available as stock are 750-mg vials, which are reconstituted for injection
using 10 ml of water for each vial. How many millilitres will be administered
to deliver the correct dose?

(b) Drug K is available as a powder in an ampoule containing 500 mg. This
is reconstituted with 10 ml of water for injection. What dose of Drug K is
delivered in an injection of 25 ml?

12.5   (a) A patient has been prescribed 180 mg of Drug L, which is supplied as an
oral solution containing 100 mg in 5 ml. What volume of the oral solution is
required?

(b) A patient has been prescribed 25 mg of Drug M, which is supplied as an oral
solution containing 10 mg in 5 ml. What volume of the oral solution is required?

(c) A patient has been prescribed 1.5 g of Drug N, which is supplied as an oral
solution containing 200 mg in 5 ml. What volume of the oral solution is
required?

(d) An ampoule of Drug P contains 40 mg in 4 ml. A patient requires 35 mg as
an intravenous bolus. What is the correct volume to be administered?

12.6   What are the concentrations in mg per ml of the solution of Drugs L, M, N and
P in check-up question 12.5(a) – (d) above?

12.7   A patient requires 35 units of Actrapid® insulin subcutaneously. Actrapid® is
available in a 10-ml vial containing 100 units per ml.

(a) How many units of Actrapid® are there in a 10-ml vial?

(b) What volume is required to administer the correct dose?

12.8   A vial of Drug Q contains a total volume of 50 ml with a concentration of 5 mg
per ml.

(a) What is the total dosage of Drug Q in one vial?

(b) For a patient requiring 125 mg of Drug Q intravenously as a slow infusion what is the total volume to be administered?

12.9 Benzylpenicillin is prescribed at a dose of 100 mg per kg daily. On admission a child is weighed and found to be 30 kg. (a) What is the total daily dose required for this child? (b) This daily dose is to be administered in 4 equal 6-hourly doses by intravenous infusion. What is the 6-hourly dose?

12.10 Drug R is given by slow intravenous infusion at a dose of 250 mg/kg daily in 3 equal 8-hourly doses. (a) What is the total daily dosage required for a neonate who weighs 4.0 kg? (b) What is the 8-hourly dose?

12.11 The drug vincristine is a chemotherapy drug prescribed for some children's cancers at a recommended dose of 1.5 mg per m^2. What is the correct dose of vincristine for a child with a BSA of 0.6 m^2?

12.12 One of the results of Example 12.8 is included in the following table of common infusion rates. Complete the table, giving the infusion rates to the nearest millilitre per hour.

Fluid	Volume infused	Time	Infusion rate
Dextrose 5%	1000 ml	8 hours	125 ml/h
Dextrose 5%	500 ml	4 hours	
Sodium chloride 0.9%	1000 ml	6 hours	
Sodium chloride 0.9%	1000 ml	12 hours	
Sodium chloride 0.9%	500 ml	6 hours	
Metronidazole 5 mg/ml	100 ml	1 hour	
Dextrose 5%	500 ml	4 hours	
Hartmann's solution	500 ml	3 hours	

12.13 A 9-year-old child is to receive an infusion of 30 ml of a metronidazole preparation, to be administered over 15 minutes. At what rate in ml/h should the infusion pump be set?

12.14 A volume of 1000 ml of dextrose 5% is to be given by intravenous infusion over 10 hours.

(a) What is the correct rate for the infusion to be delivered, in ml per hour?

(b) Find the drop rate (drops per minute) using a standard giving set.

12.15 A volume of 500 ml of dextrose 5% is to be given by intravenous infusion over 6 hours.

(a) What is the correct rate for the infusion to be delivered, in ml per hour?

(b) Find the drop rate (drops per minute) using a standard giving set.

(Continued)

(Continued)

12.16   One unit of blood has been prescribed for a patient and is to be infused over 4 hours. The unit contains 480 ml of blood.

(a) What is the correct rate for the infusion to be delivered, in ml per hour?

(b) Find the drop rate (drops per minute) using a standard giving set.

12.17   The drop rate required for an infusion is calculated to be 48 drops per minute. This rate is checked by counting the number of drops over 20 seconds, using a watch with a seconds-hand. If 18 drops are counted in this time, is this correct? too low? or too high?

12.18   (See Example 12.10 earlier in the chapter) A pregnant woman is anaemic and unable to tolerate oral iron preparations; she has been prescribed 800 mg of intravenous infusion iron dextran. The iron dextran is available as stock in 10-ml ampoules containing 50 mg/ml and is to be added to 500 ml of sodium chloride 0.9% and infused over 4 hours.

(a) What is the volume of iron dextran required to provide the dose of 800 mg?

(b) When this is added to the 500 ml of sodium chloride, what is the total volume of fluid?

(c) What is the infusion rate to administer the iron dextran and sodium chloride preparation over 4 hours?

PERCENTAGES

13

OBJECTIVES

In a practical healthcare context the practitioner should be able to:

- explain the meaning of percentages and recognize their usefulness for comparing proportions
- use informal methods or a calculator to express a proportion as a percentage
- recall and use common equivalences between fractions, decimals and percentages
- interpret concentrations expressed in percentage form
- use informal methods or a calculator to calculate a percentage of a given number or quantity
- express a change in a number or measurement as a percentage increase or decrease
- increase or decrease a number or quantity by a given percentage

Percentages are so widely-used for expressing proportions, for comparing statistics and for describing increases and decreases, that they can turn up in almost any context, not least in a variety of situations in the context of healthcare. This chapter covers all the knowledge and skills related to percentages with which any numerate professional should be confident.

SPOT THE ERRORS

Identify any obvious errors in the use of percentages in the following ten statements.

1 The condition of 90% of patients with acute sore throat resolves within 7 days without antibiotics; this means 90 resolutions without antibiotics per 100 patients.

2 A total of 38 out of 200 hospital staff travel to work by bicycle; this proportion of the hospital staff is 19%.

3 A dose of 40% of 400 mg is the same as $\frac{1}{4}$ of 400 mg, which equals 100 mg.

4 If 62.5% of an infusion has been delivered, then 37.5% of it is still to be infused.

5 As a percentage the fraction $\frac{1}{3}$ is 33.3% to three significant digits.

6 A weight of 0.4 kg = 40% of a kilogram = $\frac{2}{5}$ of a kilogram.

7 The recommended dose of Drug A for an adult patient is 200 mg per day. This is reduced to 75% for an elderly patient. So for this patient the recommended dose is 150 mg per day.

8 The recommended dose of Drug B for an adult patient is 200 mg per day. This is reduced by 25% for an elderly patient. So for this patient the recommended dose is 50 mg per day.

9 Two minutes after a brisk walk an adult's pulse rate reduces from 125 beats per minute to 100 beats per minute, so it has reduced in this time by 25%.

10 A solution of lidocaine hydrochloride 0.2% w/v contains 0.2 g of lidocaine per 100 ml of the solution, which is 2 g per litre.

Are the errors you have spotted potentially serious in medical health practice?

(errors identified on page 168)

What is a percentage?

Percent means 'per hundred'. The symbol for 'percent' is %. This is another example of the pervasive 'per' (see Chapter 12). So, for example, to say that 23% of a population are over the age of 65 years means that 23 *per* 100 are over the age of 65. Sometimes we say '23 in a hundred', or '23 out of a hundred'. This means that the proportion of those over 65 is $^{23}/_{100}$ of the entire population. A percentage is therefore essentially just a fraction with 100 as the denominator. So, 23% also means 23 hundredths. An important principle is that 100% means the whole number, the whole population, or the whole quantity being considered. So, since $100 - 23 = 77$, we can conclude that because 23% of the population are over the age of 65, then 77% of the population are *not* over the age of 65.

Example: what is 20%?

20 per cent is:

- 20 per 100
- 20 in 100
- 20 out of a 100
- 0.20
- $^{20}/_{100}$
- $^{1}/_{5}$

EXAMPLE 13.1

The proportion of patients suffering from clostridium difficile who respond positively to treatment with metronidazole within 14 days is found to be 92%. This means that the proportion of patients found to respond positively within 14 days is 92 per 100. As a fraction this proportion is $^{92}/_{100}$ of the total number of patients treated.

An implication of this data is that 8% do not respond positively within 14 days. This means 8 per 100 patients are found not to respond positively, which, as a fraction, is $^{8}/_{100}$ of those treated.

So a percentage is easily expressed as an equivalent fraction with 100 as the denominator. If, in a survey, 15% of those sampled responded 'no' to a question, 40% responded 'yes', and 45% responded 'don't know' then these results expressed as fractions are: $^{15}/_{100}$ said 'no', $^{40}/_{100}$ said 'yes', and $^{45}/_{100}$ said 'don't know'. If appropriate, these fractions can then be cancelled down to their simplest forms:

$$15\% = 15 \text{ per } 100 = {}^{15}/_{100} = {}^{3}/_{20}$$

$$40\% = 40 \text{ per } 100 = {}^{40}/_{100} = {}^{2}/_{5}$$

$$45\% = 45 \text{ per } 100 = {}^{45}/_{100} = {}^{9}/_{20}$$

ERRORS IDENTIFIED

The obvious errors are Statements 3, 8 and 9.

Statement 3

The percentage 40% is not the same as the fraction $1/4$. It is equal to $40/100$, which is equivalent to $2/5$. So 40% of 400 mg is $2/5$ of 400 mg = 160 mg.

Statement 8

Compare the correct Statement 7, which uses the phrase 'reduced to'. Statement 8 uses the phrase 'reduced by'. The different prepositions are hugely significant in understanding what is intended. Reducing by 25% of 200 mg means reducing by 50 mg. So the daily dose of 200 mg is reduced by 50 mg, to 150 mg. Yes, this is the same outcome as in Statement 7! Reducing something *to* 75% is the same as reducing it *by* 25%.

Statement 9

The pulse rate reduces by 25 beats per minute. As a fraction of the 125 beats per minute, this reduction is $25/125$, which equals $1/5$, or 20%. A reduction (or an increase) expressed as a percentage is always a percentage of the starting value, not of the reduced (or increased) value.

The errors in Statements 3 and 8 illustrate the potential serious implications of not understanding instructions that include percentages for calculating doses. Dosages of drugs for very elderly patients or for young children are sometimes prescribed as a proportion of the normal adult dose, and this proportion may be expressed as a percentage. It is obviously essential for the well-being of particularly vulnerable patients such as these that the correct proportion of the normal adult dose is calculated. Statement 8 illustrates the importance of reading instructions carefully and paying attention to the subtle use of prepositions in mathematical statements.

(now continue reading from page 167)

What is the point of using percentages?

By relating everything to 100, percentages give us a standard way of expressing a proportion of a number or quantity, thus making comparisons and our sense of the size of a proportion much easier. For example, few of us would know at a glance which of Year 1 or Year 2 has the higher proportion in these statements:

- In Year 1 a general practice recorded that 237 of the 423 patients over the age of 70 had received the influenza vaccination.
- In Year 2 the same practice recorded that 278 of the 471 patients over the age of 70 had received the influenza vaccination.

By contrast, if we are told that in Year 1 the proportion receiving the vaccination was 56% and that in Year 2 it was 59% then we know immediately that a higher proportion was achieved in Year 2.

How do you express a proportion as a percentage?

To express a proportion as a percentage all we need to do is to express it as an equivalent fraction with 100 as the denominator. If the denominator is already 100 or a multiple of 100 this is very easy!

EXAMPLE 13.2

(a) When 100 in-patients were asked whether they were satisfied with the care they received in hospital, 87 replied that they were. What percentage is this? This proportion of 87 out of 100 ($^{87}/_{100}$) is equal to 87%. This means that 87% said they were satisfied.

(b) A total of 18 out of 200 hospital staff walk to work; this proportion of the hospital staff is equivalent to 9 out of 100, which is 9%.

(c) EMLA® cream for topical anaesthesia contains two active ingredients, lidocaine and prilocaine. Each gram of cream contains 25 mg of lidocaine and 25 mg of prilocaine. Because 1 g = 1000 mg, the proportion of each of the two active ingredients is 25 in 1000, or (dividing by 10) 2.5 in 100, which is 2.5%.

Example 13.3 below provides some more examples where it is very easy to express the proportion as hundredths and thus as a percentage.

EXAMPLE 13.3

(a) So far $^1/_2$ of a preparation has been infused. Because $^1/_2$ is equivalent to $^{50}/_{100}$, the proportion of the preparation that has been infused is 50%.

(b) If $^1/_4$ of the preparation has been infused then, because $^1/_4$ is equivalent to $^{25}/_{100}$, the proportion that has been used is 25%.

(c) In part (b) above, $^3/_4$ of the preparation has not been infused, which is equivalent to $^{75}/_{100}$. As a percentage, the proportion that has not been infused is 75%.

Some equivalences to remember

$^1/_2 = 50\%$

$^1/_4 = 25\%$, $^3/_4 = 75\%$

$^1/_{10} = 10\%$

$^1/_5 = 20\%$, $^2/_5 = 40\%$

$^3/_5 = 60\%$, $^4/_5 = 80\%$

$^1/_{20} = 5\%$

If you don't know the equivalences in Example 13.3 already, learn them! Another well-known percentage is 10%, which is a proportion of 1 in 10, or $^1/_{10}$. This is because $^1/_{10} = ^{10}/_{100} = 10\%$. Most people seem to know that 10% means the same thing as a tenth. It's easy to remember. The danger is that people forget that this is a special case and think, for example, that 7% is a seventh. It isn't: 7% is $^7/_{100}$!

The examples in the box illustrate that if the proportion is a fraction with a denominator that divides exactly into 100 (that is, 2, 4, 5, 10, 20, 25, 50) then it is very easy to express it as a percentage. For example, a proportion of 1 in 5 can be expressed as the fraction $^1/_5$, which (multiply top and bottom by 20) is equivalent to $^{20}/_{100}$, which is 20%. Similarly, a proportion of 6 in 25 can be expressed as the fraction $^6/_{25}$, which (multiply top and bottom by 4) is equivalent to $^{24}/_{100}$, which is 24%.

EXAMPLE 13.4

(a) There are 52 females out of a total of 80 employees in a hospital department. What percentage is this?

The proportion of female employees is $^{52}/_{80}$, which (by cancelling 4) in its simplest form is $^{13}/_{20}$. Multiply top and bottom by 5, to get the denominator to 100, giving $^{65}/_{100}$. This means that 65% of the employees are female.

(b) To pass a clinical mathematics examination a healthcare student has to score at least 63 marks out of a possible 70 marks. What is the pass mark expressed as a percentage?

A mark of 63 out of 70 is $^{63}/_{70}$ of the marks available. This simplifies to $^9/_{10}$ (cancelling 7). To get the denominator to 100, we multiply top and bottom by 10, giving the equivalent fraction $^{90}/_{100}$, which is 90%. So the pass mark is 90%.

(a)

(b)

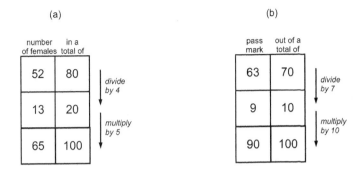

Figure 13.1   Expressing a proportion as a percentage (Example 13.4)

Figure 13.1 illustrates what we are doing in Example 13.4. These diagrams are an extension of the four-box format for solving proportionality questions that we used in Chapter 12.

In Example 13.4(a) we start with the given information: 52 females in a total of 80. We need to change this to an equivalent proportion in a total of 100. First we simplify the proportion by dividing by 4, to give us the second row. This now says the proportion is equivalent to 13 females in a total of 20. Then multiplying by 5, we get the bottom row: 65 females in a total of 100. This gives us the percentage as 65%.

In Example 13.4(b) we start with the given information: the pass mark is 63 out of a total of 80. We need to change this to an equivalent mark out a total of 100. First we simplify the proportion by dividing by 7, to give us the second row. This now says the pass mark is equivalent to 9 marks out of a total of 10. Then multiplying by 10, we get the bottom row: a pass mark of 90 out a total of 100. This gives us the percentage as 90%.

So, as we did in Chapter 12, we encourage the reader to exploit the obvious multiplication and division relationships in expressing proportions as percentages. Remember the target is always to get the proportion expressed as something in 100, or per 100, or out of 100.

Sometimes, particularly when the total number in the given data is not a factor or a multiple of 100, then there is no obvious way of doing this. Example 13.5 shows a failsafe method for expressing proportions as percentages in such cases.

EXAMPLE 13.5

Data for a group of hospitals for one particular year indicated that out of 64 patients who had received operations on the subarachnoid space of the brain there had been 11 deaths within 30 days of the procedure. What is this proportion expressed as a percentage?

(Continued)

(Continued)

The proportion of 11 out of 64 has to be converted to an equivalent proportion out of 100. Figure 13.2 shows how this might be done in two steps, going from 'per 64' to 'per 100' via 'per 1'. The given data (11 per 64) is entered into the first row. These numbers are then divided by 64 (the total number involved) to give the 1 in the right column. On a calculator 11/64 = 0.172 to 3 significant digits. This is saying effectively that the proportion of deaths is 0.172 patients per 1 patient. We then multiply this by 100 to get the number per 100, which is 17.2, as shown in the bottom row. So, the proportion expressed as a percentage is 17.2%.

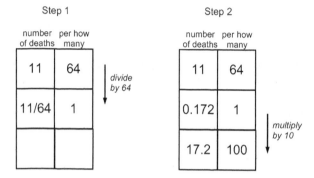

Figure 13.2   From 'per 64' via 'per 1' to 'per 100' (Example 13.5)

How do percentages relate to decimals?

The easiest mathematical procedures in this chapter are to change proportions between percentages and decimals! Because a percentage is 'so many hundredths' to change a decimal into a percentage, we simply move the decimal point two places to the right. This is just like changing an amount of money expressed in pounds into pence. Take, for example, £0.25. This is 25p, or 25 hundredths of a pound, which is 25% of a pound. So, in the same way, 0.25 of a litre is $^{25}/_{100}$ of a litre, which by definition is 25% of a litre. Similarly:

0.05 kg = 5% of a kilogram

0.8 litres (= 0.80 litres) = 80% of a litre;

0.375 g = 37.5% of a gram.

This principle also means that if you already know the decimal equivalent of a fraction, then you also know the percentage equivalent. For example, if you remember that $^3/_8$ = 0.375, then you know immediately that as a percentage $^3/_8$ = 37.5%.

Of course, it is just as easy to change a percentage into a decimal, by using the inverse process and hence moving the decimal point two places to the left. For example: 78% means $^{78}/_{100}$ or 78 ÷ 100, which equals 0.78 as a decimal, because dividing by a hundred just moves the decimal point two places to the left. So, using this principle:

35% = 0.35

7% = 0.07

12.5% = 0.125

Some more to remember

$^1/_3$ = 0.333 = 33.3%

$^2/_3$ = 0.667 = 66.7%

$^1/_8$ = 0.125 = 12.5%

$^3/_8$ = 0.375 = 37.5%

$^5/_8$ = 0.625 = 62.5%

$^7/_8$ = 0.875 = 87.5%

EXAMPLE 13.6

In a healthcare context, percentages such 0.5% and 0.05% are seen sometimes on the labels of various preparations. What are these percentages expressed as decimals? What are they as fractions?

To express as a decimal, 0.5% = 0.5/100 = 0.005.

As a fraction $^{0.5}/_{100}$ is simplified to $^1/_{200}$ (multiply top and bottom by 2).

This means 1 part in 200.

To express as a decimal, 0.05% = 0.05/100 = 0.0005.

As a fraction 0.05/100 is simplified to $^1/_{2000}$ (multiply top and bottom by 20).

This means 1 part in 2000.

How does a percentage express a concentration?

The percentage 0.9% is seen frequently in reference to a saline preparation, sodium chloride 0.9% w/v, where it refers to the concentration of the solution. The key to understanding this is the 'w/v' that often follows the percentage on the label of a solution. This is shorthand for 'weight by volume' and the convention in a healthcare context is that, unless otherwise specified, the weight is in grams and the volume is in millilitres.

So the 0.9% in 'sodium chloride 0.9% w/v' means more than just '0.9 parts per 100'; it means specifically: 0.9 *grams* of sodium chloride per 100 *millilitres* of the solution. Hence the concentration is $^{0.9}/_{100}$ g/ml. Now,

Weight by volume (w/v)

'% w/v' means 'grams per 100 millilitres'.

For example, 5% w/v means '5 g per 100 ml'.

reader, you require a little concentration yourself! Here are eight different ways of saying the same thing:

- the concentration is 0.9% w/v
- the concentration is 0.9 grams per 100 millilitres
- the concentration is $^{0.9}/_{100}$ g/ml
- expressed as a decimal the concentration is 0.009 g/ml
- this is equivalent to 9 milligrams per millilitre
- the concentration $^{0.9}/_{100}$ g/ml can be simplified to $^{9}/_{1000}$ g/ml
- this means 9 g in 1000 ml
- this is equivalent to 9 g per litre.

EXAMPLE 13.7

(a) A patient is to receive an infusion of a solution of sodium bicarbonate 8.4% w/v. What is the concentration of sodium bicarbonate in this solution in mg/ml?

The 'w/v' indicates that 8.4% here means 8.4 g per 100 ml. So the concentration is $^{8.4}/_{100}$ g/ml. Expressed as a decimal this concentration is $8.4 \div 100 = 0.084$ g/ml.

(b) A proprietary mouthwash contains chlorhexidine digluconate 0.06% w/v. What is the concentration of chlorhexidine digluconate in this preparation in micrograms per ml?

The 'w/v' indicates that 0.06% here means 0.06 g per 100 ml. So the concentration is $^{0.06}/_{100}$ g/ml. Expressed as a decimal this concentration is 0.0006 g/ml. This is equivalent to 0.6 milligrams per ml. (See Chapter 6 for converting milligrams to micrograms.)

EXAMPLE 13.8

(a) What weight of potassium chloride is there in a pre-prepared 500-ml bag of potassium chloride 0.3% (w/v)?

The concentration is 0.3 g of potassium chloride in 100 ml of the preparation. Multiplying by 5, this is equivalent to 1.5 g in 500 ml.

(b) How much dextrose is there in 30 ml of dextrose 10% w/v?

The concentration is 10 g of dextrose per 100 ml. Dividing this by 10, we get 1 g in 10 ml. Multiplying by 3 gives us 3 g in 30 ml.

(c) How much sodium chloride (in milligrams) is there in 500 ml of sodium chloride 1.8% w/v?

The concentration is 1.8 g of sodium chloride in 100 ml of solution. Multiplying by 5, in 500 ml of solution there will be 1.8 × 5 = 9 g.

Some labels will indicate that the concentration is given v/v (volume by volume) or w/w (weight by weight). The most familiar v/v example for some of us may be a wine bottle label, indicating, say, 12.5% alcohol. Pure alcohol is itself a liquid and is therefore most conveniently measured by its volume. The 12.5% here means that the concentration of alcohol in the wine is 12.5% v/v. So, there would be a volume of 12.5 ml of alcohol in a volume 100 ml of wine. Because 12.5% is equal to $\frac{1}{8}$ the concentration can also be expressed as 1 ml of alcohol in 8 ml of this wine.

EXAMPLE 13.9

(a) Some pre-injection swabs contain chlorhexidine acetate BP 0.5% w/v and isopropyl alcohol 70% v/v. Because chlorhexidine acetate is a solid it is measured by its weight, so the concentration of this chemical is given as w/v; the concentration 0.5% w/v represents 0.5 g per 100 ml, or 5 g of chlorhexidine acetate per litre. By contrast isopropyl alcohol, a liquid, is measured by volume, so it is more convenient to give the concentration as v/v; the concentration of 70% v/v means 70 ml per 100 ml, which is equivalent to 700 ml of isopropyl alcohol per litre.

(b) EarCalm® spray is a proprietary preparation for treating mild otitis externa; the label indicates that it contains acetic acid 2% w/w. The w/w indicates that the concentration in this spray is given as weight by weight. This means 2 g of acetic acid in 100 g of the preparation. This is equivalent to 0.02 g (20 mg) of acetic acid in 1 g of the spray.

How do you calculate a percentage of a number or quantity?

The answer we give to this question is: it all depends! For people who are confident in handling percentages and have at their fingertips the common equivalences between percentages and fractions and decimals, how they tackle a particular percentage calculation will depend on the numbers involved. This is comparable to our approach to proportionality questions in Chapter 12. We could just give you a rule that would apply to every question; but you would not show the kind of understanding and confidence with numbers that we are aiming for if you simply applied the same rule every time and overlooked the obvious relationships between the numbers involved. So we have five suggestions for different approaches that might be exploited for you to engage with.

Suggestion 1: Use the fraction equivalent to the percentage

EXAMPLE 13.10

The adult dosage of Drug C is 80 mg daily. For a 9-year-old child this daily dosage is reduced to 75% of the adult dosage. What is the reduced daily dosage?

We have to calculate 75% of 80 mg. Since 75% = $^3/_4$ the reduced dosage must be $^3/_4$ of 80 mg, which is 60 mg. (A quarter is 20 mg, so three-quarters is 60 mg.)

Suggestion 2: Use proportionality, remembering that the 'whole amount' is 100%.

The key to this approach is to start by writing the number or quantity that corresponds to 100%.

EXAMPLE 13.11

(a)   After 8 hours of a 12-hour infusion, 67% of a preparation of 1000 ml should have been infused. What volume is this?

We have to calculate 67%, given that 100% is 1000 ml. Figure 13.3(a) shows the proportionality between the numbers here. The obvious way of getting from numbers in the first column to those in the second is by multiplying by 10. So, the volume that should have been infused is 670 ml.

(b)   The adult dosage of Drug D is 25 mg daily. For a 12-year-old child this daily dosage is reduced to 90% of the adult dosage. What is the reduced daily dosage?

We have to calculate 90%, given that 100% (the full adult dose) is 25 mg. Figure 13.3(b) shows the proportionality between the numbers here. An obvious relationship is that you get from the first column to the second by dividing by 4. So the required dose is 90/4 = 45/2 = 22.5 mg.

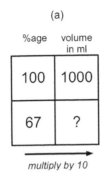
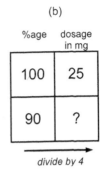

(a)

%age   volume
        in ml

100	1000
67	?

multiply by 10

(b)

%age   dosage
        in mg

100	25
90	?

divide by 4

Figure 13.3 Using proportionality to find (a) 67% of 1000 ml; (b) 90% of 25 mg (Example 13.11)

Suggestion 3: Exploit the easiness of finding 10%

This is remarkably easy and effective method! Say, we need to find 35% of some number or quantity. We can easily write down 10% (by dividing by 10). Double this and we get 20%. Halve the 10% and we get 5%. Add up the results for 10%, 20% and 5%, and we get 35%!

Ten percent

It is easy to remember that 10% is equal to a tenth. Use this as a starting point for working out other percentages informally.

EXAMPLE 13.12

Trials of Drug E indicate that 35% of 280 patients responded positively. How many patients is that?

We start with: 10% of 280 = 28

Double this: 20% of 280 = 56

Halve 10%: 5% of 280 = 14

Add 10%, 20% and 5%, we get 35% = 28 + 56 + 14 = 98 patients.

EXAMPLE 13.13

What volume of alcohol is there in 150 ml of wine with concentration 12.5% v/v?
We have to calculate 12.5% of 150 ml.

10% of 150 ml = 15 ml.

Halve this to get 5% = 7.5 ml.

Halve this to get 2.5% = 3.75 ml

Add 10% and 2.5% to get 12.5%: 15 + 3.75 = 18.75 ml of alcohol.

Suggestion 4: Change the percentage to a decimal and multiply

(See Chapter 9 for multiplications with decimal numbers.)

EXAMPLE 13.14

The usual infusion rate of maintenance fluids for an infant weighing 12 kg is 45
ml/h over 24 hours. A particular infant of this weight is prescribed 80% of this
rate. What is 80% of 45 ml/h?

80% of 45 = 0.80 × 45 = 0.8 × 45 = 36.

So the infusion rate is set to 36 ml/h.

If the numbers are more difficult than in Example 13.14, use a calculator.

EXAMPLE 13.15

It is found that 65% of cases of conjunctivitis resolve without treatment by day
five. If this proportion was determined in a sample of 240 cases, how many of
these resolved by day five?

We have to find 65% of 240, so the calculation required is 0.65 × 240, which on
a calculator gives the result 156.

(Note: you may have been taught that the calculation required here is 65 × 240 ÷ 100.
That's correct. It just seems a bit lazy to us to ask the calculator to divide by 100. So,
effectively we have done that first by changing the 65% to 0.65.)

Suggestion 5: If a calculator is required, use the percentage key (if it has one)

Some basic calculators have a percentage key (labelled %). If you have one, you will need to work out how to use it, because the procedure varies. On one calculator, for example, to find 65% of 240 we enter 65 × 240 and then press the % key, to get the result 156. Using the percentage key on a calculator is without doubt the laziest option – and the least interesting!

How do you express a change as a percentage increase or decrease?

One of the commonest uses of percentages in all walks of life is to express increases and decreases. By relating the increase or decrease to the starting value as a percentage we get a much clearer idea of the relative size and significance of the change.

EXAMPLE 13.16

(a) The cost of a pack of 60 soluble paracetamol tablets has been reduced from £5 to £4. What percentage reduction is this?

The actual reduction is £1. We have to express this as a percentage of the original price of £5 (not the reduced price £4). As a fraction 1 in 5 is $^1/_5$, which is equivalent to 20%. So the price has been reduced by 20%.

(b) An adult female patient's pulse rate is recorded at 2 pm as 65 beats per minute. The patient becomes unwell and her temperature rises. At 6 pm her pulse rate has increased to 100 beats per minute. What is the increase from 2 pm to 6 pm expressed as a percentage?

The increase is 35 beats per minute. We have to express this as a percentage of the starting value, 65 (not the increased value of 100). Following the process in Example 13.5, to express 35 as a percentage of 65, we first divide it by 65 (on a calculator, 35 ÷ 65 = 0.54 to two decimal places) and then multiply by 100, to get 54%. So there has been a 54% increase in the patient's pulse rate.

How do you increase or decrease a number or quantity by a given percentage?

This is the final process you might possibly need that involves percentages: increasing by or decreasing by a given percentage. We simply provide two examples.

Example 13.17 uses a percentage decrease and Example 13.18 a percentage increase.

EXAMPLE 13.17

(Compare spot the errors statement 8)

The recommended dose of Drug F for an adult patient is 150 mg per day. This is reduced by 20% for an elderly patient.

So for this patient the reduction to the recommended daily dose is 20% of 150 mg, which is $^1/_5$ of 150 mg = 30 mg. This is the reduction. So the reduced daily dose is 150 − 30 = 120 mg.

Note that there are two steps here: (i) find the 20% and then (ii) subtract this from the starting value. But we could do this in one step! Because the starting value is the 100%, by reducing this by 20% we must get to 80%. So we could just calculate 80% of the original dose of 150 mg: 80% of 150 mg = 0.8 × 150 mg = 120 mg.

EXAMPLE 13.18

A patient has been prescribed 250 mg per day of Drug G. Following a review it is recommended that this be increased by 20%. What is the increased daily dosage?

The increase must be 20% of 250 mg, which equals $^1/_5$ of 250 mg = 50 mg. This is the increase. So the increased daily dosage is 250 + 50 = 300 mg.

Consideration of percentage increases introduces a surprising idea: that we can have a percentage over 100%. This seems strange at first, because we have talked about 100% as representing the whole amount from which a proportion is to be taken. But if a quantity increases from a starting value that we call 100%, then the increased value will be greater than 100%. Calculations with percentages greater than 100% are no different from those we have been doing so far in this chapter.

So in Example 13.18 there were two steps: (i) find the 20% and then (ii) add this to the starting value. Because the starting value is the 100%, by increasing this by 20% we now have 120%. This means we could do Example 13.18 just by calculating 120% of the original dose of 250 mg: 120% of 250 mg = 1.2 × 250 mg = 300 mg.

13.1 (a) In Example 13.2(a), 87% of in-patients reported that they were satisfied. What percentage did not?

(b) In Example 13.2(b), 9% of the staff walked to work. What percentage did not walk to work?

13.2 Express the following as percentages:

(a) 7 in 50

(b) 150 per 1000

(c) 24 out of 25

(d) 1 in 8

(e) 60 out of 90

(f) $3/5$

(g) $73/100$

(h) $68/200$

(i) $1/30$

(j) 1p in £100

13.3 Records of children with acute otitis media show that 72 of 120 children were better within 24 hours without antibiotics. Express this proportion as a percentage.

13.4 Records of patients with acute rhinosinusitis show that 95 of 120 cases resolved within 14 days without antibiotics. Use a calculator and the method of Example 13.5 to express this proportion as a percentage.

13.5 Express the concentration of lidocaine 0.2% w/v in:

(a) g per 100 ml

(b) g per litre

(c) milligrams per ml

13.6 A gel contains metronidazole 0.8% w/v. Express the concentration in:

(a) g per 100 ml

(b) g per litre

(c) milligrams per ml

13.7 Isopropyl alcohol is registered as an antimicrobial, bactericide, fungicide and virucide, and is widely used for cleaning purposes. Isopropyl alcohol 99.9% v/v can be used, for example, for cleaning non-disposable medical devices. What do you understand by this percentage?

13.8 EMLA® cream is a lidocaine/prilocaine 5% w/w oil-in water emulsion. The two active ingredients (lidocaine and prilocaine) together constitute 5% by weight of the cream.

(a) How many milligrams of active ingredients are there per 100 mg of cream?

(b) Express this concentration as mg per gram.

13.9 Aciclovir is an antiviral agent used for the treatment of herpes simplex virus infections of the skin. How much of this antiviral agent is contained in a 2-gram tube of aciclovir 5% w/w cream?

(Continued)

(Continued)

13.10 Calculate:

(a) 80% of 200 mg   (b) 75% of 500 ml   (c) 90% of 50 ml

13.11 The adult dosage of Drug H is 120 mg daily. For an 8-year-old child this daily dosage is reduced to 70% of the adult dosage. What is the reduced daily dosage?

13.12 A little puzzle: find a number A such that A% of 20 is equal to 20% of A.

13.13 How many millilitres of alcohol are there in a 150-ml glass of wine with strength 14% v/v?

13.14 Drug J is supplied as a solution with concentration 2% w/v in 20-ml ampoules. What is the total dosage of Drug J in one ampoule?

13.15 The normal recommended total daily dose of Drug K is 100mg/kg. For an elderly patient the dose is to be reduced to 75% of the normal recommended total daily dose. What total daily dose is required if the elderly patient's weight is 60 kg?

13.16 The number of patients seen with influenza over the winter months by doctors at a general practice surgery reduces from 500 one year to 425 the next. What is the percentage reduction?

13.17 The price of 250 g of a proprietary brand of Drug L increases from £3.75 to £4.05. What is the percentage increase?

13.18 Most babies lose some weight after birth, but careful clinical assessment and evaluation of feeding is advised when weight loss exceeds 10%. A newborn baby who weighed 3.7 kg on birth is found to weigh 3.2 kg five days after birth. What percentage weight loss is this?

13.19 (a) Three weeks after pancreatic surgery an adult male patient is discharged from hospital; at this stage his weight has decreased by 20% from his admission weight of 80 kg. What is his weight on discharge?

(b) Six months later the patient has recovered well and his weight has increased by 20% from what it was on discharge from hospital. What is his weight now?

MISCELLANEOUS MATHEMATICS 14

OBJECTIVES

In a practical healthcare context the practitioner should be able to:

- interpret inequality signs ($<$, $>$, $\leq$ and $\geq$)
- substitute values correctly into algebraic formulas
- understand square roots
- use the formula for estimating body surface area
- use a variety of graphs and charts to extract data
- use a nomogram to read off an approximate value for body surface area
- use the formula for body-mass index
- understand percentiles and the median value of a set of numerical data
- calculate the mean of a set of numerical data
- do simple calculations involving moles and molar concentration

This chapter contains a range of mathematical material that may be encountered in a number of healthcare situations. Understanding this material will enable the practitioner to make sense of the professional context in which they work.

SPOT THE ERRORS

Identify any obvious mathematical errors in the following 11 statements.

1   Following healthcare guidance for a severe gastro-intestinal tract infection which states, 'Admit if T > 38.5 °C and WCC > 15', a patient with temperature 39 °C and white cell count of 16 should be admitted.

2   For two measurements, a and b, the formula $m = (a + b)/2$ gives the value m of the midpoint between a and b. When $a = 120$ and $b = 60$, $m = 90$.

3   Using the formula $T_F = 1.8T_C + 32$ to convert a temperature in degrees Celsius to degrees Fahrenheit, when $T_C = 38$, $T_F = 1.8 \times 38 + 32 = 1.8 \times 70 = 126$.

4   The square root of 6 ($\sqrt{6}$) is 3.

5   A formula for estimating body surface area for a person of height h metres and weight w kg is BSA $= \sqrt{(hw/3600)}$ square metres; if $hw = 1600$ then the BSA $= 0.667$ m^2.

6   Using the section of the (simplified) nomogram given in Figure 14.1, the approximate body surface area of a patient with height 180 cm and weight 73 kg is 1.91 m^2.

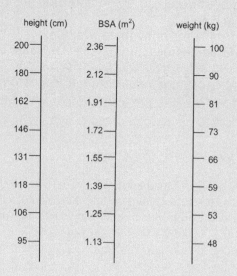

height (cm)	BSA (m^2)	weight (kg)
200	2.36	100
180	2.12	90
162	1.91	81
146	1.72	73
131	1.55	66
118	1.39	59
106	1.25	53
95	1.13	48

Figure 14.1   Section of a nomogram for finding approximate body surface area

7 In the formula for calculating the body-mass index for an adult, BMI = w/h^2, w kilograms is the person's weight, h metres is the person's height and h^2 stands for $h \times h$.

8 A BMI greater than 30 for most adults is categorized as obese. Using the data provided in the section of a BMI table in Figure 14.2 an adult of height 1.68 m weighing 87 kg is obese.

weight (kg)

height (m)	80	81	82	83	84	85	86	87	88	89
1.80	25	25	25	26	26	26	27	27	27	27
1.78	25	26	26	26	27	27	27	27	28	28
1.76	26	26	26	27	27	27	28	28	28	29
1.74	26	27	27	27	28	28	28	29	29	29
1.72	27	27	28	28	28	29	29	29	30	30
1.70	28	28	28	29	29	29	30	30	30	31
1.68	28	29	29	29	30	30	30	31	31	32
1.66	29	29	30	30	30	31	31	32	32	32
1.64	30	30	30	31	31	32	32	32	33	33
1.62	30	31	31	32	32	32	33	33	34	34

Figure 14.2   Section of a body-mass index (BMI) table

9 The weight of a 3-month-old infant is at the 80th percentile for children of that age. This means the infant's weight is 80% of the average weight of children of that age.

10 A patient's pulse rate taken at 4-hourly intervals is recorded as 66, 70, 72, 69 and 73 beats per minute. The mean of these readings is 70 beats per minute.

11 The molecular mass of sodium chloride is given as 58.5. This means that if 58.5 g of sodium chloride were dissolved in a litre of water, the concentration would be 1 mole per litre.

Are the errors you have spotted potentially serious in medical health practice?

(errors identified over the page)

ERRORS IDENTIFIED

The obvious errors are Statements 3, 4 and 9.

Statement 3

In the calculation of $1.8 \times 38 + 32$ the multiplication has precedence over the addition and must be done first. (Precedence of operators and brackets are explained in Chapter 7.) So, $1.8 \times 38 + 32$ is understood to mean $(1.8 \times 38) + 32$ which equals $68.4 + 32 = 100.4$. This tells us that a temperature of 38 °C corresponds to 100.4 °F. Although Fahrenheit temperatures are not used in clinical settings, we have used this example to illustrate an important point about understanding formulas. Anyway, the temperatures used here could refer to the weather in Seville in July.

Statement 4

Finding the square root of 6 means finding the number which when *squared* (multiplied by itself) equals 6. This is not 3, because $3 \times 3 = 9$, not 6. The square root of 6 cannot be written down exactly as a decimal number, but, using a calculator with a square root key, we find that $\sqrt{6}$ is approximately 2.45. Checking: $2.45^2 = 2.45 \times 2.45 = 6.0025$, which is 6.00 to 3 significant digits.

Statement 9

This is a complete misunderstanding of a percentile. To say that the weight of a 3-month-old infant is at the 80th percentile for children of that age means that the lightest 80% of children of that age will have a weight less than or equal to that weight.

These errors are all significant in healthcare practice, even though as they stand they are not life-threatening. The error in Statement 3 might be indicative of a practitioner's potential for wrongly using a simple algebraic formula for calculating the value of an important variable related to a patient's health. The error in Statement 4 might indicate that a practitioner confuses squaring with doubling and finding a square root with halving. This could lead, for example, to errors in calculating body-mass index and in using the formula for body surface area. Understanding percentiles is important in monitoring an individual against the norms of the population; for example in Statement 9 (corrected) the percentile is an indication that the child is well above average weight for children of the same age.

What are inequality signs all about?

In this section, we just want to make sure you are familiar with the use and meanings of inequality signs ($<$, $>$; $\leq$ and $\geq$).

Inequality signs

$a < b$ means a is less than b

$b > a$ means b is greater than a

$a \leq b$ means a is less than or equal to b

$b \geq a$ means b is greater than or equal to a

An indicator for assessing confusion in a patient might be 'score < 8' on a particular mental test. This simply means 'a score less than 8'; in other words, a score of 7, 6, 5, 4, 3, 2, 1 or 0. The symbol '$<$' means 'less than' or 'fewer than'.

Some primary care advice for the treatment of shingles is to 'treat with aciclovir if age > 50 years and time of diagnosis ≤ 72 h of rash'. This statement uses the symbols $>$ and $\leq$, which are simply abbreviations for 'greater than' and 'less than or equal to', respectively. Mainly in mathematics we are concerned with things being equal or equivalent, so we get used to using the equals sign ($=$). But there are times when we wish to state that something applies over a range of values; and then these inequality signs may be useful. In the statement above, 'age > 50 years' means simply 'age greater than 50 years'; and 'time of diagnosis ≤ 72 h of rash' means that the time at which the diagnosis was made was 'less than or equal to' 72 hours of the rash appearing.

EXAMPLE 14.1

Blood pressure is recorded in mmHg (millimetres of mercury) with two measurements: the systolic pressure (SP), which is the pressure in the arteries when the heart contracts, and the diastolic pressure (DP), which is the pressure in the arteries when the heart rests between contractions. Hypertension (high blood pressure) is recognized when one or both of the following is recorded by the practitioner: SP > 140, DP > 90.

This would include: (a) a patient with blood pressure of 160/80 (the usual way of referring to SP $= 160$ and DP $= 80$), because SP > 140, even though DP < 90; (b) a patient with blood pressure 135/105, because DP > 90, even though SP < 140; (c) a patient with blood pressure 170/110, because both SP > 140 and DP > 90.

Sometimes we need to make statements about a range of values lying *between* two values. These can also be expressed concisely using inequality signs. For example, a forecast that the temperature today ($t\ °C$) will lie between 7 °C and 15 °C could be abbreviated to: $7 < t < 15$. This means that both $7 < t$ (7 will be less than the temperature) and $t < 15$ (the temperature will be less than 15) are being forecast. This could also be written as $15 > t > 7$. Note that $<$ and $>$ do not include the end-points of the range, but $\leq$ and $\geq$ do.

'Lies between'

$a < b < c$ means a is less than b, and b is less than c.

$c > b > a$ means c is greater than b, and b is greater than a.

Both mean that b lies between a and c.

EXAMPLE 14.2

If T is an adult's temperature measured in °C to one decimal place, then one classification gives 'normal' as $36.5 \leq T \leq 37.5$ and 'fever' as $37.5 < T \leq 38.3$.

In each of these statements T has to satisfy two inequalities. So, $36.5 \leq T \leq 37.5$ means that both $36.5 \leq T$ and $T \leq 37.5$ must be true. Hence for 'normal' T can take any value from 36.5 (including 36.5) up to and including 37.5. Similarly, $37.5 < T \leq 38.3$ means that both $37.5 < T$ and $T \leq 38.3$ must be true. Hence for 'fever' T can take any value between 37.5 and 38.3, including 38.3.

What is there to know about algebraic formulas?

As an example, there is a formula that is sometimes used in healthcare with children aged 4 to 10 years to predict quickly the likely internal diameter in millimetres (*d mm*) for an uncuffed endotracheal (ET) tube required for a child of a given age. For age *n* years, the formula is: $d = n/4 + 4$.

In essence a formula expresses the mathematical relationships between two or more *variables*. A variable is a quantity or measurement that can theoretically take different values within some range. In the above example, the variables are the predicted diameter of the tube, measured in mm, and the age of the child, measured in years. The diameter is restricted to various values from 2 to 10.5 mm, because the diameters of available ET tubes lie in this range. We are told that the age of the child can take different values from 4 to 10.

In algebra we use letters to represent variables: like the *d* and the *n* in the formula above. Variables are often dependent on each other so that when one changes the others change. A formula enables us to track such changes, by finding the value of one variable – called the *dependent* variable – when we know the values(s) of the other(s) – called the *independent* variable(s).

In the example above, the dependent variable is *d* and the independent variable is *n*. The diameter of the ET tube in mm (*d*) is dependent on the age of the child in years (*n*). We can then *substitute* actual values of the independent variable(s) and find the corresponding value of the dependent variable. For example, for a child aged 8 years, $n = 8$ and so $d = 8/4 + 4 = 2 + 4 = 6$. So the formula predicts that an ET tube with internal diameter of 6 mm will be required.

Here are a few things to note about algebraic formulas.

- Often a multiplication sign in front of a letter (a variable) or a bracket will be omitted, so for example $2 \times n$ will be written as $2n$, $h \times w$ will be written as hw, and $5 \times (y + 2)$ will be written as $5(y + 2)$. See, for example, the formula in *Spot the errors* Statement 3, where $1.8T_c$ means 1.8 multiplied by the value of T_c.

- Division is usually represented by a forward stroke (/), as, for example the $n/4$ in the formula above for ET tube diameter. Division can also be represented by a horizontal line, as shown in Figure 14.3, where it means: divide the value of the expression above the line by 9.
- Brackets in a formula always indicate which calculations must be done first. A horizontal line used for division acts like a bracket around everything written above the line. For example, in Figure 14.3, if $T_F = 99$, the very first calculation to be done is the 99 – 32 within the brackets. This is then multiplied by 5, and then the result of the whole calculation above the line is divided by 9.
- Multiplication and division always take precedence over addition and subtraction, other than when brackets indicate otherwise. Failure to use this principle was the error in *Spot the errors* Statement 3. The multiplication by 1.8 has to be done *before* the addition of the 32. In the ET tube diameter formula above, the '$n/4 + 4$' does *not* mean n divided by '$4 + 4$'. It means divide n by 4 and *then* add 4. The division must be done first.

$$T_C = \frac{5(T_F - 32)}{9}$$

Figure 14.3   An algebraic formula for converting temperatures in °F to °C

EXAMPLE 14.3

(a) Use the formula $d = n/4 + 4$ to predict the ET tube diameter that might be required for a child age 6 years.

In this case, $n = 6$, so $d = 6/4 + 4 = 1.5 + 4 = 5.5$. The predicted tube diameter is 5.5 mm.

(b) A formula proposed for predicting ET tube length in centimetres (L) for a child aged n years (n in the range 4 to 10) is $L = n/2 + 13$. What length of tube is predicted for a child age 10 years?

Substituting $n = 10$, the formula gives $L = 10/2 + 13 = 5 + 13 = 18$. The predicted length is 18 cm.

(c) Use the formula in Figure 14.3 to convert 97 °F to °C.

Substituting $T_F = 97$, the expression above the line becomes 5(97 – 32) which equals $5 \times 65 = 325$. So $T_C = 325/9 = 36.1$ (to 3 sig. fig.). So 97 °F is equivalent to 36.1 °C.

What are square roots?

The square of a number n is the result of multiplying n by n. This is written n^2 and read as 'n squared'. In Chapter 1, for example, we showed how 100 (= 10 × 10) can be written as 10^2 (ten squared). In a similar way, 20^2 (twenty squared) = 20 × 20, which equals 400, and 0.2^2 = 0.2 × 0.2, which equals 0.04.

Finding the square root of a number is the inverse process of finding a square. So, because the square of 20 is 400, then the square root of 400 is 20. Because the square of 0.2 is 0.04, then the square root of 0.04 is 0.2. The symbol for square root is $\sqrt{\ }$. So we would write $\sqrt{400}$ = 20 and $\sqrt{0.04}$ = 0.2, reading these as 'the square root of 400 is 20' and 'the square root of 0.04 is 0.2'.

One example of where it is necessary to calculate a square root is when using the formula (see below) for estimating body surface area. Finding a square root is usually a job for a calculator with a square root key, since most square roots do not work out exactly as decimal numbers. This key might be labelled $\sqrt{\ }$ or (particularly on a scientific calculator) $\sqrt{x}$. For example, to find $\sqrt{40}$, we would enter the number 40, press the square root key, and the result would be displayed, to however many digits the calculator can display. On one calculator we got $\sqrt{40}$ = 6.3245553. To check this we could multiply this number by itself and expect to get back to 40 (allowing for the possibility of a small rounding error). Not all basic calculators have square root keys.

You may recognize certain numbers as 'perfect squares'; these are the squares of whole numbers. For example, you may know that 4 is 2^2, that 9 is 3^2, that 16 is 4^2, that 25 is 5^2, and so on. So, you also know: $\sqrt{4}$ = 2, $\sqrt{9}$ = 3, $\sqrt{16}$ = 4, $\sqrt{25}$ = 5, and so on. You can use these to get a sense of what size of answer you might expect when finding a square root.

EXAMPLE 14.4

The formula for body surface area (explained below) gives the result $\sqrt{3.5}$ m² (square metres) for a man of height 175 cm and weight 72 kg. We would expect the result of this to be a bit less than 2 m², because 3.5 is less than 4 and we know $\sqrt{4}$ = 2. A calculator gives the result $\sqrt{3.5}$ = 1.87 (to 3 significant digits).

What is the formula for estimating body surface area (BSA)?

Average BSA

To give you some idea what to expect: most BSAs range from about 0.25 m² for an average neonate to about 2.5 m² for a large adult male.

We saw in Chapter 12 that the dosage of some drugs is based on an individual's body surface area (BSA). A number of different formulas have been devised for estimating body surface area. This is because the relationship between body surface area and other variables is not an exact one, and the best that any formula can do is to give us an estimate. Some do this better than others in

particular ranges of the variables. The formula most often used, the Mosteller formula, is, fortunately, the simplest:

$A = \sqrt{(hw/3600)}$

where h centimetres is the height of the individual, w kilograms is their weight, and A
square metres is the body surface area (BSA).

The formula tells us to multiply h by w, divide the answer by 3600, and then calculate the square root of the result. This will almost certainly be a job for a calculator.

EXAMPLE 14.5

The recommended dosage of Drug A is 2.5 mg/m². Calculate the dose for a
9-year-old girl with height 1.20 m and weight 45 kg.

The Mosteller formula requires h to be in centimetres, so the first step is to
convert the girl's height to 120 cm. We now have $h = 120$, $w = 45$. So $hw = 120 \times$
$45 = 5400$. Next we divide by 3600: $5400/3600 = 54/36 = 3/2 = 1.5$. Note that we
have chosen to do these particular calculations mentally, because they happen
to be quite accessible. Using a calculator, the estimated BSA is $\sqrt{1.5} = 1.225$ m²
(rounded to 3 decimal places).

The dose required for this BSA is $2.5 \times 1.225 = 3.0625$ mg, which might then be
rounded to 3.1 mg.

What is a nomogram?

First, let's be clear that a nomogram is not another unit of weight like the milligram or
kilogram! The suffix 'gram' here refers to something written or drawn, as in anagram
or diagram. A nomogram is any kind of graphical representation of the relationship
between some variables in which the value of the dependent variable is found by a
simple graphical construction. The most common example for healthcare practitioners is a nomogram used to find an estimate for a person's BSA from the values of their
height and weight, without the need to do any calculations.

To illustrate how this kind of nomogram works we have provided a simplified
version of a section of a BSA nomogram in Figure 14.1, earlier in the chapter. To
use this you just identify the point on the left-hand scale representing the person's
height and the point on the right-hand scale representing their weight and connect
these with a ruler. The point where the ruler crosses the central scale is then read
off as an estimate for the BSA.

Check now that Statement 6 in the *Spot the errors* section at the start of this chapter
is correct. Place a ruler on Figure 14.1 so that it joins 180 on the height scale to 73 on
the weight scale. You should find that it crosses the central scale at the point marked as
1.91, indicating a BSA estimate of 1.91 m².

EXAMPLE 14.6

Use Figure 14.1 to estimate the BSA for a 12-year-old of height 146 cm and weight 48 kg.

Join 146 on the height scale to 48 on the weight scale using a ruler. The ruler crosses the central scale at the point 1.39, so the estimated BSA is 1.39 m².

BSA nomograms can be accessed online or in medical reference books. Some nomograms are specifically designed for estimating BSA for children. We suggest that you access one or two examples of BSA nomograms. For example, do an online search for 'West BSA nomogram' or 'Lentner 1981 BSA nomogram'.

Use the West BSA nomograms, for example, to estimate the body surface area of a child of height 116 cm and weight 38 kg. This will require finding the point on the height scale between, say, 110 and 120, that represents 116; and the point on the weight scale between, say, 35 and 40, that represents 38. The Mosteller formula gives an estimate for the BSA as $\sqrt{(116 \times 38/3600)} = 1.107$ (to 3 decimal places). Do not be surprised if the estimate you get from a nomogram is slightly different – nor if different nomograms give slightly different results. Estimating body surface area is not an exact science and various nomograms are based on different formulas.

What is the formula for body-mass index (BMI)?

The body-mass index (BMI) is a means of judging whether a person's weight is appropriate for their height. The formula used to calculate the body-mass index (BMI) for an adult is:

$$BMI = w/h^2$$

where w kilograms is the person's weight and h metres is the person's height.

BHF categories

The British Heart Foundation uses these categories for BMI:

BMI > 30   very overweight

25 < BMI ≤ 30   overweight

18.5 ≤ BMI ≤ 25   healthy

BMI < 18.5   underweight

http://www.bhf.org.uk/bmi/home.html

Notice that in this formula the height (h) is in metres, whereas in the BSA formula above the height (h) was in centimetres. The formula tells us to divide w by the square of h (that is $h \times h$). For example, for a man with $w = 70$ (kilograms) and $h = 1.80$ (metres), the BMI is $70/(1.80^2) = 70/3.24 = 21.6$ (rounded to 1 decimal place).

This index is used to give an indication of whether a person's weight is in a healthy range, or too high or too low for their height. A BMI of 21.6 lands this man safely in the healthy category (BMI from 18.5 to 25, inclusive). We should note that there are limitations to interpreting a body-mass index in this way. The categorizations given here are not appropriate, for example, for pregnant women, men of very athletic build or children.

The table given in Figure 14.2, earlier in the chapter shows BMIs for a small range of heights and weights. A full table can be downloaded from the British Heart Foundation (BHF) website: http://www.bhf.org.uk/bmi/home.html.

Notice that if the value of h stays the same the BMI increases in proportion to the weight. Reading the row for height 1.70 m in the table in Figure 14.2 we can see how the BMI changes for a man of height 1.70 m as his weight increases from 80 kg to 89 kg. At 80 kg, his BMI is 28, which is in the overweight category. At a weight of 83 kg he has moved to BMI = 29. At a weight of 86 kg his BMI is 30. At a weight of 89 kg, he has moved to a BMI of 31 and is now (BMI > 30) categorized as very overweight (obese).

By scanning the values down a column, we can see also that that if the weight is fixed and the height *decreases* then the BMI *increases*. So, for example, a woman weighing 82 kg is only just overweight if she is 1.80 m tall (BMI = 25), but very overweight (obese) if she is only 1.62 m tall (BMI = 31).

EXAMPLE 14.7

Using the formula BMI = w/h^2, we can calculate the BMI for a man of height 182 cm and weight 60 kg. Note that the height must first be written in metres, as 1.82 m. The BMI = $60/(1.82^2)$ = 60/3.3124 = 18.1 (to one decimal place). This means that this man is underweight.

Consulting the table of BMI values on the BHF website and looking down the column for height 1.82 metres, we can see that this man will require a weight of 62 kg in order to move just into the healthy category, with a BMI of 19.

Figure 14.4 is an example of the kinds of graphical representation of data that are commonly used in healthcare practice. Make sure you can interpret graphs like this! The

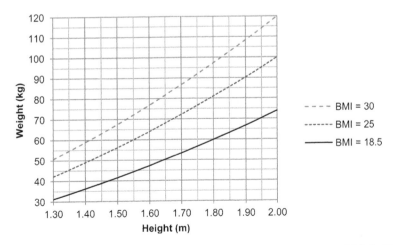

Figure 14.4 Graph showing heights and weights giving BMIs of 18.5, 25 and 30

horizontal and vertical axes represent respectively the variables 'height in metres' and 'weight in kilograms'. As an example, follow the vertical line up from 1.70 m on the height axis. This meets the curve drawn for BMI = 18.5 just below the horizontal line that meets the weight axis at 55 kg (halfway between 50 and 60) – say, at about 54 kg. This means that a person of height 1.70 m has to weigh about 54 kg to achieve a BMI of 18.5, which is the lower limit for 'healthy'. Continue moving up the 1.70-metre line and we see that it meets the next curved line (for BMI = 25) at a height of about 72 kg. This is the boundary between healthy and overweight.

Continuing upwards, the 1.70-metre line meets the top curved line (for BMI = 30) at a weight of about 87 kg. This is the boundary between overweight and obese.

So we see that the three curved lines divide the area of the graph into four sections:

1 below the BMI = 18.5 curve, underweight;
2 between the BMI = 18.5 and BMI = 25 curves, healthy;
3 between the BMI = 25 and BMI = 30 curves, overweight;
4 above the BMI = 30 curve, very overweight (obese).

EXAMPLE 14.8

Using Figure 14.4 we can categorize the following individuals: (a) a man of height 1.75 m and weight 82 kg is overweight; (b) a woman of height 1.57 m and weight 43 g is underweight.

What are percentiles?

Percentiles: an example

Line up all the numbers in a set of numerical data in order from the smallest to the largest. The value that is 30% of the way along the line is the 30th percentile.

'For the weights of baby boys in the UK aged 22 weeks the 75th percentile is 8.1 kg.' We will explain the meaning of this sentence. It refers first of all to a *population*: in this case, baby boys in the UK aged 22 weeks. It refers secondly to a *variable* that has a value for each member of the population: in this case, their weight in kilograms. We now imagine that we get hold of all the members of this population, strap them in their carrycots and then line them up in order from the lightest baby on the left to the heaviest baby on the right. Now start at the beginning of the line on the left, walk 75% (three-quarters) of the way along the line and stop. The weight of the baby you are now standing beside (8.1 kg, of course) is the 75th percentile!

What it means, therefore, to say that the 75th percentile is 8.1 kg is that the lightest 75% of the babies in this population weigh 8.1 kg or less. It also means that the 25% heaviest babies weigh 8.1 kg or more. (Note: there may be lots of babies whose weights are recorded as 8.1 kg, hence the use of both '8.1 kg or less' and '8.1 kg or more'.

Percentiles help us to relate the value of the variable in question for an individual to the values across the whole population. For this same population, the 25th percentile is 7 kg. This means that the lightest 25% of 22-week baby boys weigh 7 kg or less; and the heaviest 75% weigh 7 kg or more. So, if 22-week baby Jack weighs 7.3 kg, we can see from these percentiles that Jack is not in the lightest 25% for his age (he is over 7 kg), nor in the heaviest 25% (he is under 8.1kg). Jack's weight lies between the 25th and 75th percentiles, so his weight is fairly average and there should be no concern about it.

The table in Figure 14.5 gives the values of a range of percentiles for this particular population.

Percentile	0.4th	2nd	9th	25th	50th	75th	91st	98th	99.6th
Weight (kg)	5.5	6.0	6.5	7.0	7.5	8.1	8.75	9.3	10

Figure 14.5 Values of various percentiles for the weights of UK baby boys aged 22 weeks

Consider the 50th percentile, 7.5 kg. This tells us that if we walked 50% of the way along the line the baby we would be standing next to would weigh 7.5 kg. This value, the 50th percentile – the weight of the baby bang in the middle of the line – is called the *median* weight of the population. The median is a kind of average, very handy for giving a representative value of a variable for large populations.

The median value

The median value of a set of numbers or measurements is the 50th percentile: the value of the item in the middle if all the items in the set are arranged in order.

EXAMPLE 14.9

(a) Baby Luke is 22 weeks old and weighs 6.2 kg. How does this compare with other boy babies of Luke's age? The table in Figure 14.4 shows that Luke's weight is somewhere between the 2nd and 9th percentiles. We could reckon that his weight puts him in roughly the bottom 5% for weight amongst baby boys of his age.

(b) Baby Hercules is 22 weeks old and weighs 10.1 kg. This puts Hercules above the 99.6th percentile for weight. The 99.6th percentile is 10 kg. This means up to 0.4% of baby boys of this age weigh more than this – that's only 4 in 1000, or 1 in 250.

The data in Figure 14.5 was taken from the World Health Organization (WHO) Boys UK-WHO growth chart 0–4 years, available (at the time of writing), along with similar charts for girls, on the Royal College of Paediatrics and Child Health (RCPCH) website:

http://www.rcpch.ac.uk. These charts include data for weight, lengths and head circumference. We recommend that readers access these charts, read carefully the advice about how to interpret them and work out how we have obtained the values quoted above. Note that 'percentiles' are sometimes called 'centiles'.

A simplified version of the growth chart for the weights of boys aged 2 to 10 weeks, showing just 9th, 50th and 91st percentiles is given in Figure 14.6. This shows, for example, that at 8 weeks the 50th percentile weight (median weight) of baby boys is about 5.4 kg. The 9th and 91st percentiles at 8 weeks are about 4.5 kg and 6.3 kg; this means that all but the lightest 9% and the heaviest 9% of boy babies at the age of 8 weeks will have weights in the range 4.5 to 6.3 kg.

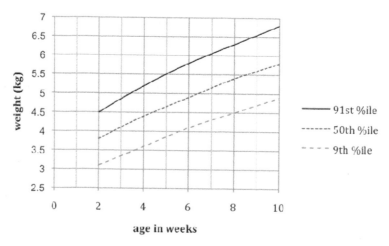

Figure 14.6 Extract from growth chart for weights of boys aged 2 to 10 weeks

What is the mean of a set of data?

An average is a representative value for a set of data. It is used essentially for three purposes.

1 First, an average value enables us to make comparisons between two populations or sets of data. For example, we might say: 'on average men are taller than women'.
2 Second, an average value enables us to compare one member of the population with the whole population. For example, we might say: '3-month-old baby Elin is lighter than average for baby girls of her age'.
3 Third, an average value enables us to see an underlying trend as the values of a variable go up and down. For example, we might say: 'this patient's average temperature over the last 12 hours has been 38.5 °C'.

There are a number of different types of average that are used in various contexts. For the first two examples above, with large sets of data, the average that would be used is the *median* value, which, as we have explained above, is the 50th percentile.

To find the mean of a set of values

(a) Find the total of all the values in the set.

(b) Divide by the number of values in the set.

Another common type of average is the *mean* (technically it is the arithmetic mean) of a set of data. Imagine that a group of people sitting round a table put onto the table all the cash they are carrying and then share it out equally between them. The amount that each would get is the mean amount of cash that they were carrying. This scenario helps us to understand how a mean average value is calculated. You add up the total of all the cash available and then divide it equally by the number of people around the table.

Similarly, to find the mean average of six readings of a patient's temperature during a 12-hour period, you would add up all the readings and divide the total by 6.

EXAMPLE 14.10

(a) A patient's pulse is taken at four 4-hour intervals and recorded as: 98, 93, 86, and 90 beats per minute. The mean pulse rate over this period is (98 + 93 + 86 + 90)/4 = 367/4 = 92 beats per minute (rounded to the nearest whole number).

(b) The scores of the men in a numeracy test on a healthcare training programme were 78%, 54%, 99%, 92% and 62%. The scores of the women were 85%, 80%, 79%, 85%, 64% and 93%. Overall who did better?

The mean score for the 5 men was (78 + 54 + 99 + 92 + 62)/5 = 385/5 = 77%.

The mean score for the 6 women was (85 + 80 + 79 + 85 + 64 + 93)/6 = 486/6 = 81%.

Overall, the mean scores suggest that the women did better than the men. But both groups need to do better!

What are moles and molar concentration?

Understanding the ideas explained in this section may not be necessary in all health-care contexts. But, since practitioners who actually read labels and instructions are likely occasionally to come across concentrations that use moles and millimoles, we assume you would like to be able to make some sense of them. It is also a good excuse to give you some more practice in handling the mathematics of proportionality!

In previous chapters we have mostly expressed concentrations of solutions as weight by volume (w/v), such as mg per ml. In chemistry what is often more significant is the *number* of particles (molecules) per unit of volume. For example, chemically it is

Moles and molecular mass: an example

The molecular mass of potassium sulphate is 174.

So 1 mole of potassium sulphate will weigh 174 grams.

Some molecular masses

Calcium chloride	147
Glucose	180
Potassium chloride	74.5
Potassium sulphate	174
Sodium bicarbonate	84
Sodium chloride	58.5
Sodium phosphate	358

more useful to know *how many* molecules of calcium chloride have been dissolved in 100 ml to produce a solution of calcium chloride 10% than knowing that the weight of calcium chloride in 100 ml of the solution is 10 g. But the numbers are huge. Counting at the rate of two per second it would take about 60 trillion years to reach the number of molecules in 1 gram of calcium chloride

So, pharmacists will sometimes express the number of particles dissolved in a solution using numbers called *moles* (abbreviation, mol). A mole is a number, a very big number. It is approximately equal to 6×10^{23}; that's 6 followed by 23 zeros. Quite how this arcane number got to be chosen for this role is interesting, but not particularly relevant to our explanation. All we need to note is that the clever thing about this number is that it is chosen in a way that enables us to write the next paragraph!

The most important thing to know about counting in moles is this: if the *molecular mass* of a chemical compound is m then 1 mole of the compound weighs m grams. For example, the molecular mass of calcium chloride is 147. This means that 147 g of calcium chloride will contains 1 mole of calcium chloride molecules. The molecular mass is a way of measuring the mass of one molecule of a substance. In simple terms it tells us how many times the mass of one molecule is greater than the mass of one hydrogen atom. It can be worked out from the chemical formula for the compound, but for our purposes it can be obtained from a table of molecular masses, such as the one shown in the box.

EXAMPLE 14.11

(a) How many moles of sodium bicarbonate are there in 100 g?

The molecular mass of sodium bicarbonate is 84.

So, 84 g of this compound contains 1 mol of molecules.

So, 1 g contains 1/84 mol and 100 g contains $(1/84) \times 100$ mol.

Using a calculator, this gives us 1.19 mol of sodium bicarbonate molecules in 100 g.

(b) How many moles of calcium chloride are there in 10 g?

The molecular mass of calcium chloride is 147.

So, 147 g of this compound contains 1 mol of molecules.

So, 1 g contains 1/147 mol and 10 g contains $(1/147) \times 10$ mol.

Using a calculator, this gives us 0.068 mol of sodium bicarbonate molecules in 10 g. This will usually be expressed as 68 millimoles; this is abbreviated to 68 mmol. The prefix 'milli' means 'a thousandth of', just as in millilitre and milligram.

Concentrations can therefore be expressed in terms of moles and millimoles. For example, we might come across a concentration of 2 mol/litre (2 moles per litre) or 500 mmol/litre (500 millimoles per litre). How do we relate these to w/v concentrations?

Moles (mol) and millimoles (mmol)

1 mol = 1000 mmol

1 mmol = 0.001 mol

EXAMPLE 14.12

(a) How many moles of sodium bicarbonate are there in a 10-ml injection of sodium bicarbonate 8.4%?

The concentration of sodium bicarbonate 8.4% is 8.4 g per 100 ml.

This is equivalent to 84 g per litre.

Now the molecular mass of sodium bicarbonate is 84. This means that 84 g is equivalent to 1 mol. The concentration is therefore 1 mol/litre. This neat result is not a fluke: this is precisely why the concentration of 8.4% is used for this particular chemical!

A concentration of 1 mol/litre is 1000 mmol/litre. This means that a 10-ml syringe of sodium bicarbonate 8.4% will deliver 10 millimoles.

Similarly, a 50-ml syringe will deliver 50 millimoles.

(b) A concentration of 4.2% is used for a sodium bicarbonate intravenous injection.

This means that there is half as much sodium bicarbonate in a litre as there is in the 8.4% concentration. So the concentration of sodium bicarbonate 4.2% is 0.5 mol/litres, or 500 mmol/litre.

So a 10-ml syringe of sodium bicarbonate 4.2% will contain 5 mmol.

(c) A concentration of 1.26% is used for a sodium bicarbonate intravenous infusion.

This is 1.26 g per 100 ml, which is equivalent to 12.6 g per litre.

Since 84 g is equivalent to 1 mol, then 1 g is equivalent to 1/84 mol. So, 12.6 g is equivalent to $(1/84) \times 12.6$ mol = 0.15 mol = 150 mmol.

So the concentration is 150 mmol/litre.

This concentration also gives 'neat' results. For example, 100 ml contains 15 mmol, so an infusion rate of 100 ml/h would deliver 15 mmol/h.

Blood glucose levels might be recorded in both mmol/litre and mg per 100 ml. The next example illustrates how these measurements are related.

EXAMPLE 14.13

The normal blood glucose level for non-diabetic individuals is about 4 mmol/litre. What is this in mg per 100 ml?

The molecular mass of glucose is 180; so 1 mol is equivalent to 180 g.

So 4 mmol (0.004 mol) is equivalent to $0.004 \times 180 = 0.72$ g.

So the normal blood glucose level is about 0.72 g per litre.

This is equivalent to 720 mg per litre, or 72 mg per 100 ml.

For readers who wish to pursue this topic, some further examples of calculations involving moles and molar concentrations are given in Chapter 15.

HAVE A CHECK-UP

14.1 Find a whole number n for which both these statements are true: $10 < n < 15$ and $12 > n > 7$.

14.2 Here's a formula that could be used to find the drop rate per minute (d) for an infusion of blood, given the volume of infusion in ml (v) and the time of infusion in minutes (t): $d = 15v/t$. Use this formula to find d when $v = 500$ and $t = 240$.

14.3 Use the formula in Figure 14.3 to convert a temperature of 100 °F to °C.

14.4 (a) Find the values of $\sqrt{9}$, $\sqrt{90}$, $\sqrt{900}$, $\sqrt{9000}$, $\sqrt{90\,000}$ and $\sqrt{900\,000}$. Use a calculator with a square root key, when necessary, and give answers to three significant digits.

(b) Now, without using a calculator, write down the values of $\sqrt{9\,000\,000}$ and $\sqrt{90\,000\,000}$.

14.5 (a) Use the simplified nomogram in Figure 14.1 to read off an estimate for the body surface area of a woman of height 146 cm and weight 48 kg.

(b) Compare this reading with the estimate obtained using the Mosteller formula for BSA.

14.6 The recommended dosage for the weekly injection of doxorubicin for a child with leukaemia is 30 mg/m². What would be the weekly dosage for a 3-year-old boy whose weight is 16.5 kg and whose height is 0.93 m?

14.7   Use the graph in Figure 14.4 and the BHF categories to categorize the following adults:

(a) Amir who is 1.82 m tall and weighs 85 kg;

(b) Bess who is 1.70 m tall and weighs 50 kg;

(c) Corinne who is 1.43 m tall and weighs 45 kg.

14.8   Use a calculator and the BMI formula to find the BMI for a man of weight 90 kg and height 171 cm. Give the result to the nearest whole number. Is this a healthy weight for this man?

14.9   Calculate the BMI for a woman of height 4 feet 8 inches and weight 10 stone 1 pound.

14.10   (a) Use Figure 14.6 to read off the 91st percentile weight for boys aged 3 weeks. What does this tell you about the heaviest 9% of boys of this age?

(b) Baby Harry is 5 weeks old and weighs 3.1 kg. What does Figure 14.6 tell you about Harry's weight?

(c) What is the median weight for boys aged 6 weeks?

14.11   The temperature at 3 pm in a hospital ward in a week in the summer is recorded each day as follows: 25 °C, 26 °C, 28 °C, 29 °C, 26 °C, 24 °C, 23 °C. What was the mean temperature at 3 pm that week?

14.12   (a) The molecular mass of potassium chloride is 74.5. What is the weight of 1 mole of potassium chloride?

(b) What weight of potassium chloride is equivalent to 35 mmol?

(c) Express the concentration of sodium chloride 0.9% as mmol/litre. The molecular mass of sodium chloride is 58.5.

(d) What concentration of sodium chloride (% w/v) would be equivalent to 1 mol/litre? (Compare Example 14.12 earlier in the chapter).

(e) The concentration of a solution of sodium phosphate (molecular mass 358) is given as 0.5 mol/litre. Express this concentration in g per 100 ml and hence in the form % w/v.

APPLICATION

15

OBJECTIVE

In a practical healthcare context the practitioner should be able to apply their understanding of mathematical processes, concepts and principles, appropriately, accurately and confidently, to various situations that might be encountered in practice, including:

- dosage examples
- infusion rate calculations
- fluid requirements for children
- growth charts
- molar concentrations and chemical formulas
- displacement volume
- situations involving a number of different calculations

The examples in this final chapter draw on the mathematical knowledge, skills and concepts that we have explained in previous chapters. Each example describes a healthcare situation, poses a question or questions, and provides a detailed explanation of how each question might be answered. Where appropriate we use what might be the most obvious mental or informal calculation strategies. The reader may well opt for other ways of doing the calculations involved; that's fine by us! Use whatever methods you are comfortable with. As a guide, in each example we indicate whether or not we think the calculations involved require the use of a calculator.

Reminder

Volume = dose required divided by concentration

Dosage examples

Examples 15.1 – 15.6 give you the opportunity to revisit the principles for the calculation of dosages based on concentrations, as explained in Chapter 12, and to extend your skills in handling these.

EXAMPLE 15.1

Details: A practitioner has to check the dose of a morphine sulphate injection for a patient who is in severe pain and has been prescribed 15 mg of morphine sulphate as an intravenous bolus.

The morphine is available in a 2-ml ampoule containing 10 mg per ml.

Questions: (a) What is the correct volume to be administered?

(b) Is there sufficient in the 2-ml bolus?

Calculator: Should not be needed. This is a question of proportionality (see Chapter 12) in which there are very obvious relationships between the numbers involved (such as 10 and 15) that can be exploited.

Answers: (a) The concentration of 10 mg per ml means that 1 ml contains 10 mg. The patient requires 15 mg.

The proportion 10 mg in 1 ml is equivalent to 15 mg in 1.5 ml.

So, 1.5 ml will be required.

(b) The bolus, which contains 2 ml, is sufficient to provide the 1.5 ml required.

EXAMPLE 15.2

Details: A patient requires an injection of 150 mg of disopyramide.

Disopyramide is available in 5-ml ampoules, with a concentration of 10 mg/ml.

Questions: (a) What volume should be injected?

(b) How many ampoules are required?

Calculator: Should not be needed for this level of calculations.

Answers: (a) To find the volume required, divide the dose required by the concentration: 150/10 = 15 ml.

Check: 15 ml at 10 mg/ml will contain 15 × 10 mg = 150 mg.

(b) For 15 ml a total of 3 ampoules each containing 5 ml will be required.

EXAMPLE 15.3

Details: During a hospital admission a child aged 6 years and weighing 18 kg is prescribed digoxin for an arrhythmia.

The child is to receive an initial loading dose of digoxin of 25 micrograms per kg.

This will be given as an oral elixir containing 50 micrograms per ml.

Question: What volume of the elixir should be given as an initial dose?

Calculator: Should not be needed, since the only calculations involved are multiplying by 25 and recognizing that 450 is 50 multiplied by 9.

Answer: If the initial dose is 25 micrograms/kg, then the dose for a child weighing 18 kg is 25 × 18 micrograms = 450 micrograms.

The elixir contains 50 micrograms in 1 ml.

The 450 micrograms required is 9 times 50 micrograms (see Figure 15.1 and the explanation of proportionality in Chapter 12).

So, 9 ml of elixir is required as an initial dose.

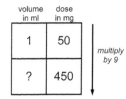

Tips

To multiply by 25: multiply by 100 and then divide by 4.

To divide by 4: halve and halve again.

Figure 15.1   In Example 15.3 the dose is proportional to the volume of elixir

EXAMPLE 15.4

Details: A premature baby born at 36 weeks weighing 2.5 kg is prescribed oral paracetamol at a dose of 20 mg/kg as a single dose, then 10 mg/kg every 6–8 hours as necessary.

A maximum of 60 mg/kg can be given in 24 hours in divided doses.

Questions: (a) What is the initial single dose required for the baby?

(b) What is the subsequent reduced dose?

(c) What is the maximum total dosage of paracetamol that this baby is able to receive in 24 hours?

(d) If the baby is given the reduced dose 3 times at 6-hourly intervals, is the total dosage within the maximum permitted?

Calculator: Should not be necessary for the multiplications by 10, 20 and 60 and the simple addition required in this calculation.

Answers: (a) The initial dose at 20 mg/kg is 20 × 2.5 = 50 mg.

(b) The reduced dose at 10 mg/kg = 10 × 2.5 = 25 mg.

(c) The maximum dose permitted within 24 hours at 60 mg/kg is 60 × 2.5 = 6 × 25 = 150 mg.

(d) After the initial dose of 50 mg, the baby is given a further 25 mg after 6 hours, 12 hours and 18 hours. The total dosage is 50 + (3 × 25) = 125 mg, which is within the 150 mg maximum.

EXAMPLE 15.5

Details: A child aged 4 years is prescribed aciclovir at a dosage of 250 mg/ m^2 by intravenous infusion every 8 hours for 5 days.

The child has height 102 cm and weight 16.5 kg.

Question: What is the amount required for each individual dose?

Calculator: Will be required if using the BSA formula to estimate the child's body surface area.

Answer: Since the dosage is given in mg/m², we have to estimate the child's body surface area. We could read this off from a nomogram or use the Mosteller formula (see Chapter 14.) We will use the formula BSA = $\sqrt{(hw/3600)}$, where h is height in cm and w is weight in kg, for which a calculator is required.

For this child the formula gives BSA = $\sqrt{(102 \times 16.5/3600)} = \sqrt{0.4675}$ = 0.684 (to 3 decimal places).

Each individual dose is 250 mg/m², so the dose for this child is 250 × 0.684 = 171 mg, to the nearest milligram.

Having just reminded you about nomograms, we will now risk confusing you by introducing *nanograms*! A nanogram is a very small unit of weight, one-thousandth of a microgram. So the relationship between nanograms and micrograms is the same as that between micrograms

Nanogram (ng)

1 ng = 0.001 micrograms

1000 ng = 1 microgram

and milligrams, and between milligrams and grams: 1 g = 1000 milligrams; 1 milli-gram = 1000 micrograms; 1 microgram = 1000 nanograms. The symbol for nanogram is ng. Example 15.6 below uses nanograms.

EXAMPLE 15.6

Details: The range of recommended daily doses of alfacalcidol for children aged 2–12 years is 15–30 ng/kg.

Alfacalcidol is available in an oral suspension with concentration 2 micrograms per ml.

Questions: (a) What volumes of the suspension provide doses within the range of recommended daily doses for a 5-year-old child of weight 20 kg?

(b) Is a volume of 0.2 ml of the suspension within this range?

(c) What dose of alfacalcidol would 0.2 ml provide?

Calculator: Not required. The questions require only simple multiplications and divisions, some cancelling of fractions and some knowledge of decimal equivalents for fractions (see Chapter 11).

Answers: (a) The lower limit of the dose range is 15 ng/kg. For a weight of 20 kg, this is a dose of $15 \times 20 = 300$ ng. The upper limit is twice this, which is 600 ng. So the range of doses is from 300 ng to 600 ng.

The suspension contains 2 micrograms per ml, which is equivalent to 2000 ng per ml.

To provide 300 ng and 600 ng, volumes of 300/2000 ml and 600/2000 ml respectively will be required.

$300/2000 = 3/20 = 0.15$ ml.

$600/2000 = 6/20 = 3/10 = 0.3$ ml.

The range of volumes of the suspension for a child of weight 20 kg is therefore from 0.15 ml to 0.3 ml.

(b) A volume of 0.2 ml lies with this range. We could write $0.15 < 0.2 < 0.3$ (see Chapter 14 for > and < symbols).

(c) A volume of 0.2 ml provides a dose of 0.2×2 micrograms = 0.4 micrograms = 400 ng.

Infusion rate calculations

The examples in this section give you the opportunity to revisit, reinforce and extend your skills in handling the calculations involving infusion rates that were explained in Chapter 12. Example 15.7 that follows involves changing an infusion rate from hours to minutes.

EXAMPLE 15.7

Details: An adult patient is prescribed a glyceryl trinitrate (GTN) infusion for pulmonary oedema.

The infusion consists of 50 mg of GTN in dextrose 5%, making a total volume of 250 ml.

The infusion rate is set at 20 ml/h.

Question: How many micrograms per minute (micrograms/min) of GTN is the patient receiving?

Calculator: Not required for a multiplication like 20×0.2; you also need to know the decimal equivalents of $^1/_5$ and $^2/_3$, and to use the latter to find 200/3.

Answer: The concentration of 50 mg of GTN in 250 ml is 50/250 mg/ml = 1/5 mg/ml = 0.2 mg/ml.

The infusion delivers 20 ml per hour.

The dosage of GTN in a volume of 20 ml is $20 \times 0.2 = 4$ mg. So the infusion delivers 4 mg per hour, which is 4000 micrograms per hour.

To express this as micrograms/min divide by 60, giving 4000/60 micrograms/min.

Cancelling 20: 4000/60 = 200/3. Since 2/3 = 0.667 (to 3 significant digits), 200/3 will equal 66.7.

The rate of delivery of GTN is 66.7 micrograms/min.

EXAMPLE 15.8

Details: A patient is started on an intravenous infusion of 1 litre of dextrose 5% at 6 am. This is set to infuse at a rate of 125 ml/h. After 4 hours the doctor reviews the patient's progress and the infusion rate is to be reduced by 33.3%.

Questions: (a) What is the total volume of dextrose 5% infused by 10 am?

(Continued)

(Continued)

(b) To what rate is the infusion reduced after the review?

(c) Following the reduction in the rate, how long will the remaining dextrose 5% take to run through?

Calculator: It might be necessary to use a calculator for parts (b) and (c).

Answers: (a) At a rate of 125 ml/h, in 4 hours the volume infused is 125 × 4 = 500 ml.

(b) A reduction of 33.3% is a reduction of a third ($^1/_3$); $^1/_3$ of 125 = $41^2/_3$ = 41.7 (approximately). So the rate is reduced to 125 – 41.7 = 83.3 ml/h.

(c) There is a volume of 500 ml still to be infused. The time required to infuse this at a rate of 83.3 ml/h is 500/83.3 = 6 hours.

Another Reminder

Infusion time = volume to be infused divided by infusion rate

In Example 15.9 below there are three variables involved in proportion to each other: the number of units of the drug, the volume of the infusion and the time of the infusion.

EXAMPLE 15.9

Details: A heparin infusion is prescribed for a patient at 1000 units/h and is to be administered using an infusion pump.

The infusion is made up of 25 000 units of heparin in dextrose 5%, making a total volume of 500 ml.

Questions: (a) How long will it take to complete the 500-ml infusion?

(b) What is the rate in ml/h that the infusion pump will be set at to deliver the 1000 ml/h?

Calculator: Should not be needed for multiplying and dividing by 25.

Answers: Figure 15.2 shows how the method of boxes we introduced in Chapter 12 for solving proportionality problems can be employed for the three variables involved here.

What we know is written in the boxes.

In the top row we know that 25 000 units correspond to 500 ml. We have to find (a) the time it should take to complete this infusion.

In the bottom row, because the rate prescribed is 1000 units/h, we know that 1000 units of heparin are to be delivered in 1 hour. We have to find (b) the volume corresponding to this number of units.

(a) The numbers in the units column show that to get from the bottom row to the top row, we multiply by 25. So, multiplying the 1 hour by 25 we get 25 hours for the time required to deliver the 25 000 units.

(b) To get from the top row to the bottom row we must divide by 25. So, dividing the 500 ml by 25 gives 20 ml as the volume that delivers 1000 units in 1 hour. Hence the rate for the infusion is 20 ml/h.

units of heparin	volume in ml	time in hours
25 000	500	?
1000	?	1

multiply by 25   divide by 25

Figure 15.2 The three variables in Example 15.9

Fluid requirements for children

In paediatric nursing it is important to monitor fluid balance. Dehydration for a sick child can lead to clinical deterioration. The normal fluid requirement over 24 hours for a child over 5 kg of weight can be calculated using this 'formula':

- 100 ml/kg for each of the first 10 kg of the child's weight
- 50 ml/kg for each of the second 10 kg
- 20 ml/kg for any additional kilograms.

Use this formula in the following three examples.

EXAMPLE 15.10

Details: Baby Fatima, a girl of 6 months, weighs 7.5 kg.

Question: What would be the normal daily fluid requirements for Fatima?

Calculator: Not required for multiplication by 100.

Answer: Fatima weighs less than 10 kg, so only the 100 ml/kg rate applies. For her weight of 7.5 kg, the daily fluid requirement is $100 \times 7.5 = 750$ ml.

EXAMPLE 15.11

Details: 5-year-old Jon weighs 22 kg.

Jon has a cardiac abnormality and requires 75% of the normal fluid requirement.

Questions: (a) What would be the normal daily fluid requirement for a child of Jon's weight?

(b) What is Jon's daily fluid requirement?

Calculator: Not required for multiplication by 10 and 100, nor for simple addition. May possibly be needed for calculating $^3/_4$ of 1540.

Answers: (a) The first 10 kg of Jon's weight at 100 ml/kg gives 1000 ml.

The second 10 kg of his weight at 50 ml/kg gives 500 ml.

The remaining 2 kg of his weight at 20 ml/kg gives 40 ml.

Two ways to find $^3/_4$ of a number

- find one quarter and then multiply by 3

- find one quarter and subtract this from the number

The normal daily fluid requirement for a child of Jon's weight is 1000 + 500 + 40 = 1540 ml = 1.540 litres.

(b) Jon's requirement is 75% of this, which is $^3/_4$ of 1540 ml.

This can be done mentally: a half of 1540 is 770, and half of this is 385.

So, $^1/_4$ of 1540 ml is 385 ml. Hence $^3/_4$ of 1540 ml is 385 × 3 = 1155 ml.

Jon's daily fluid requirement is 1155 ml or 1.155 litres.

EXAMPLE 15.12

Details: An infant with a cardiac abnormality weighs 12 kg.

The infant is prescribed 75% of normal maintenance fluids over 24 hours.

The infant is receiving an infusion amounting to 20 ml/hour of fluid.

The infant is also receiving antibiotics given in fluid form, which amount to a further 10 ml every three hours.

Questions: (a) What is this infant's total fluid requirement over 24 hours?

(b) How much fluid per hour, in addition to the infusion and antibiotics, should be given to this infant?

Calculator: Probably advisable for division by 24.

Answers: (a) Using the formula given earlier, the normal fluid requirement for an infant of 12 kg is $(100 \times 10) + (50 \times 2) = 1100$ ml, over 24 hours.

For this infant the requirement is 75% of 1100 ml = $^3/_4$ of 1100 ml.

Mentally, $^3/_4$ of 1100 = ($^3/_4$ of 1000) + ($^3/_4$ of 100) = 750 + 75 = 825.

So this infant's requirement over 24 hours is 825 ml.

(b) 825 ml over 24 hours is equivalent to 825/24 ml/h = 34.4 ml/h (rounded to 1 decimal place).

The infusion provides 20 ml per hour.

The antibiotics provide 10/3 = 3.3 ml per hour (rounded to 1 decimal place).

The total fluid intake should not exceed 34.4 ml/h.

So the amount of additional fluid this infant requires is 34.4 – (20 + 3.3) = 34.4 – 23.3 = 11.1 ml per hour. This would be rounded to 11 ml/h.

Growth charts

For the two examples that follow, you should access the child growth charts for girls 0–4 years on the website of the Royal College of Paediatrics and Child Health (RCPCH): www.growthcharts.rcpch.ac.uk. These questions reinforce the explanations of percentiles given in Chapter 14.

EXAMPLE 15.13

Details: Baby Kate, aged 12 weeks, is found to weigh 7.4 kg, to have a length of 62 cm and to have a head circumference of 42.5 cm.

Questions: (a) Approximately, what are the median values of weight, length and head circumference for girls of 12 weeks?

(b) Approximately, what are the ranges of values that lie within the 25th and 75th percentiles (centiles) for these three measurements for girls of 12 weeks?

(Continued)

(Continued)

      (c) With respect to these three measurements, how does baby Kate compare with other children of this age?

Calculator: No calculations involved.

Answers: (a) The median values are the 50th percentiles. Reading from the growth charts these are approximately: weight, 5.7 kg; length, 59 cm; head circumference, 39 cm.

      (b) The ranges from the 25th to the 75th percentile are approximately: for weight, from 5.2 kg to 6.2 kg; for length, from 58 cm to 61 cm; for head circumference, from 38.3 cm to 40 cm.

      (c) Baby Kate is well above average for all three of these measurements. Her weight puts her around the 98th percentile, so she is one of the heaviest 2% of baby girls of her age. Her length puts her around the 91st percentile, which is in the longest 9%. And her head size is around the 99.6th percentile, which is larger than all but 0.4% (4 in 1000) of baby girls of this age.

The middle 50%

Remember that for any given variable half of those in a population have values from the 25th to the 75th percentile values.

EXAMPLE 15.14

Details: The growth charts for girls 0–4 years include a weight-height to BMI conversion chart for children over 2 years. This is referred to for Megan aged 3 years (36 months), who weighs 12.7 kg and has a height of 100 cm.

Questions: (a) Convert Megan's weight and height to percentiles for girls who are 3 years of age.

      (b) Use the weight-height to BMI conversion chart to determine the percentile (centile) equivalent for Megan's body-mass index.

      (c) What does the answer to (b) mean?

Calculator: No calculator needed to read the charts.

Answers: (a) Megan is around the 25th percentile for weight and the 91st percentile for height.

(b) Follow the horizontal line from the 25th percentile on the weight axis until it meets the vertical line from the 91st percentile on the height axis. They meet on one of the sloping lines. Follow this line to the BMI axis. This indicates that Megan's BMI is at the 2nd percentile.

(c) This means that Megan's body-mass index is very low, in the bottom 2%. This is a cause for concern and may indicate malnutrition.

Molar concentrations and chemical formulas

In Chapter 14 we explained that moles and millimoles are (very large) numbers. We also explained how to use the molecular mass to calculate the number of moles or millimoles of a substance in a given weight and how to express concentrations in mol/litre or mmol/litre, and so on. Example 15.15 applies these ideas for those who wish to further their understanding.

EXAMPLE 15.15

Details: A total of 25 mmol of potassium chloride is to be added to a 1-litre infusion.

A 10-ml ampoule contains 2 g of potassium chloride.

The molecular mass of potassium chloride is 74.5.

Question: What volume should be drawn up?

Calculator: May be helpful for multiplying 25 by 0.0745.

Answer: The molecular mass tells us that 74.5 g of potassium chloride is equivalent to 1 mol, or 1000 mmol.

So 1 mmol is equivalent to 0.0745 g (dividing 74.5 by 1000).

For 25 mmol the weight of potassium chloride required is therefore 25×0.0745 g = 1.8625 g.

The concentration is 2 g in 10 ml, which is 0.2 g/ml.

So, for 1.8625 g we must draw up $1.8625/0.2 = 18.625/2 = 9.3$ ml (rounded to 1 decimal place).

In Example 15.15 we have been focussing on moles and millimoles of potassium chloride. In pharmacy, often more significant than the number of potassium chloride molecules dissolved in a solution are the numbers of separate potassium and chlorine ions. The chemical formula for potassium chloride is KCl. K stands for potassium and Cl for chlorine. This means that when dissolved in water each molecule of potassium chloride produces one potassium ion and one chlorine ion. So, in Example 15.15 the 25 mmol of potassium chloride will produce 25 mmol of potassium ions and 25 mmol of chlorine ions.

EXAMPLE 15.16

Details: One litre of sodium chloride 1.8% is to be infused.

The chemical formula for sodium chloride is NaCl, where Na stands for sodium and Cl for chlorine.

The molecular mass of sodium chloride is 58.5.

Questions: (a) What is the concentration of the infusion in mmol/litre?

(b) How many millimoles of sodium are there in the whole infusion?

Calculator: Will be required.

Answers: (a) The molecular mass tells us that 58.5 mg of NaCL contains 1 mol of molecules, or 1000 mmol.

The concentration of 1.8% tells us that we have 1.8 g in 100 ml, which is equivalent to 18 g in 1 litre.

We have to find how many mmol in 18 g, given 1000 mmol in 58.5 g.

Using the principles of proportionality, the number is $18 \times 1000/58.5 = 308$ mmol (to 3 significant digits).

So the concentration is 308 mmol/litre.

(b) Each molecule of NaCl produces 1 sodium ion. So the infusion contains 308 mmol of sodium.

Displacement volume

When a solvent is dissolved in a diluent the solvent may appear to disappear, but it still occupies space and therefore adds a little to the total volume. This is called the displacement volume. For example, 100 mg of diamorphine powder displaces 0.6 ml of water. This means that it adds 0.6 ml to the total volume when dissolved. These displacement volumes may be small, but they can be significant when dosage calculations have to be very precise, for example, when calculating doses for children. We give one example to illustrate the effect of displacement volumes.

EXAMPLE 15.17

Details: 1 g of amoxicillin displaces 0.8 ml of diluent.

200 mg of amoxicillin powder is to be reconstituted.

The resulting solution is to have a total volume of 5 ml.

Question: How much diluent must be added to the 200 mg of amoxicillin?

Calculator: Should not be necessary. Remember that to divide by 5 you can divide by 10 and then double the answer.

Answer: If 1 g (1000 mg) of amoxicillin displaces 0.8 ml, then 200 mg will displace 0.8/5 ml = 0.16 ml.

So, for a total volume of 5 ml, the volume of diluent required is only 4.84 ml. (Note that 4.84 + 0.16 = 5 and 5 − 0.16 = 4.84.)

When 4.84 ml of diluent is used to reconstitute 200 mg of amoxicillin powder, the result is 200 mg of amoxicillin in 5 ml.

If we had reconstituted the 200 mg of powder in 5 ml of diluent then the total volume would have been 5.16 ml.

Situations involving a number of different calculations

EXAMPLE 15.18

Details: A patient has a Patient Controlled Analgesia (PCA) infusion pump running. It contains 5 mg of morphine in a total of 20 ml made up with sodium chloride 0.9%.

The pump is programmed to infuse a total of 1.8 mg of morphine over 24 hours.

The PCA pump is programmed to deliver a single bolus dose of 0.5 ml as required by the patient.

Questions: (a) What is the concentration of the morphine infusion in mg/ml?

(b) What is the total volume to be delivered in 24 hours?

(c) What is the rate at which the infusion pump will be set to deliver this?

(d) What is the dosage of morphine delivered in each bolus?

(Continued)

(Continued)

Calculator: Probably not needed. Even the trickiest division here can be handled by some nifty multiplying and cancelling to get simpler equivalent ratios.

Answers: (a) A concentration of 5 mg in 20 ml is equivalent to 1 mg in 4 ml or $^1/_4$ mg in 1 ml = 0.25 mg/ml.

(b) The patient requires 1.8 mg in 24 hours. To get the volume required to deliver 1.8 mg we divide it by the concentration, giving 1.8/0.25 ml. Simplify this by multiplying both numbers by 4, giving 7.2/1 = 7.2 ml. The total volume to be delivered is 7.2 ml.

(c) To deliver 7.2 ml in 24 hours requires a rate of 7.2/24 ml/h.

Simplify this by multiplying both numbers by 10, giving 72/240 ml/h.

Cancel 24, to get 3/10 ml/h, which is a rate of 0.3 ml/h.

(d) The concentration is 0.25 mg/ml, so the 0.5-ml bolus will contain half of 0.25 mg, which is 0.125 mg.

EXAMPLE 15.19

Details: Khalid, a 65-year-old man, is admitted to hospital after becoming acutely short of breath while at home. Following assessment by the doctor Khalid is diagnosed with acute left ventricular failure and pulmonary oedema. On admission Khalid weighs 70 kg.

The doctor prescribes:

2.5 mg of morphine intravenously

80 mg of furosemide intravenously as a stat (immediate) dose

a GTN infusion of 5 micrograms/kg per minute

a dobutamine infusion of 2.5 micrograms/kg per minute

Questions: (a) The GTN infusion is prepared with 100 mg of GTN in a total volume of 50 ml. At what rate, in ml/hr, should the GTN infusion be set?

(b) The dobutamine infusion is prepared containing 500 mg in a total volume of 500 ml. At what rate, in ml/hr, should the dobutamine infusion be set?

Calculator: Probably not needed, unless you cannot handle 350 × 60 mentally.

Answers: In both questions here we follow the same route:

- find the dosage in micrograms per minute
- convert to micrograms per hour
- convert to milligrams per hour
- use the concentration to find the required volume per hour.

(a) For a weight of 70 kg a dosage of 5 micrograms/kg of GTN is 5 × 70 = 350 micrograms. So Khalid requires 350 micrograms/min.

The next step is to change the minutes to hours.

$$350 \text{ micrograms/min} = 350 \times 60 \text{ micrograms/h} = 21\,000 \text{ micrograms/h.}$$

350 × 60 mental calculation

To multiply by 60, multiply by 2 then by 3 then by 10.
350 → 700 → 2100 → 21 000

This is equivalent to 21 mg/h.

The next step is to find how many millilitres are needed to deliver 21 mg.

We are given 100 mg in 50 ml, which is 1 mg in 0.5 ml. This is a simple case of proportionality (see Chapter 12). The dose of 21 mg will be contained in 0.5 × 21 ml = 10.5 ml.

2.5 × 70 mental calculation

This is half of 5 × 70; half of 350 = 175.

The required infusion rate is 10.5 ml/h.

175 × 60 mental calculation

This is half of 350 × 60, which we found to be 21 000. Half of 21 000 is 10 500.

(b) The dosage of dobutamine for a patient weighing 70 kg is 2.5 × 70 = 175 micrograms/min.

Then 175 micrograms/min = 175 × 60 micrograms/h = 10 500 micrograms/h.

This is equivalent to 10.5 mg/h.

The concentration is 500 mg in 500 ml, which is 1 mg/ml.

The required volume is 10.5 ml/h.

EXAMPLE 15.20

Details: Acetylcysteine is available as a 10-ml ampoule containing 200 mg per ml.

A patient has been prescribed acetylcysteine at an initial dose of 150 mg/kg.

This is to be infused in 200 ml of dextrose 5% intravenously over 15 minutes.

(Continued)

(Continued)

The initial dose is followed by a continuous infusion of 50 mg/kg in 500 ml of dextrose 5% over the next 4 hours.

This is then followed by 100 mg/kg in 1 litre of dextrose 5% over 16 hours.

The patient weighs 73.5 kg.

Questions: (a) What is the initial dose of acetylcysteine in mg required for this patient? What volume of acetylcysteine in ml should be added to the 200 ml of dextrose 5% to deliver this dose? What is the required infusion rate in ml/h at which an infusion pump should be set for the initial 15-minutes infusion?

(b) What is the dose in mg of acetylcysteine required for the subsequent 4-hours infusion? What volume of acetylcysteine in ml should be added to the 500 ml of dextrose 5% to deliver this dose? What is the required infusion rate in ml/h at which the infusion pump should be set for the 4-hours infusion?

(c) What is the dose in mg of acetylcysteine required for the final 16-hours infusion? What volume of acetylcysteine in ml should be added to the 1 litre of dextrose 5% to deliver this dose? What is the required infusion rate in ml/h at which the infusion pump should be set for the 16-hours infusion?

Calculator: It might be appropriate to use a calculator here for multiplications by 73.5.

Answers: The three questions related to each of the three stages of this patient's treatment are answered in the same way.

(a) At 150 mg/kg the initial dose for a weight of 73.5 kg is $150 \times 73.5 = 11\,025$ mg (11.025 g).

The concentration in each ampoule is 200 mg per ml. We require 11 025 mg. Divide the weight by the concentration to get the volume: $11025/200 = 55.125$ ml. (This will require six 10-ml ampoules.)

Delaying rounding

Notice that as much as we can we delay rounding in these calculations until the final result, to avoid a rounding error in one calculation affecting the results of subsequent calculations. (See Chapter 8.)

The total volume to be infused is 200 ml of dextrose 5% plus 55.125 ml acetylcysteine = 255.125 ml.

This is to be infused over 15 minutes.

So the infusion rate = 255.125 ml per quarter of an hour = 255.125×4 ml per hour = 1020.5 ml/h.

This would be rounded to 1020 ml/h.

(b) At 50 mg/kg the dose for a weight of 73.5 kg is 50 × 73.5 = 3675 mg (3.675 g).

The concentration in each ampoule is 200 mg per ml. We require 3675 mg. Divide the weight by the concentration to get the volume: 3675/200 = 18.375 ml. (This will require two 10-ml ampoules.)

The total volume to be infused is 500 ml of dextrose 5% plus 18.375 ml acetylcysteine = 518.375 ml.

This is to be infused over 4 hours.

So the infusion rate = 518.375/4 ml per hour = 129.59375 ml/h. This can be rounded to 130 ml/h.

(c) At 100 mg/kg the dose for a weight of 73.5 kg is 100 × 73.5 = 7350 mg (7.350 g).

The concentration in each ampoule is 200 mg per ml. We require 7350 mg. Divide the weight by the concentration to get the volume: 7350/200 = 36.75 ml. (This will require four 10-ml ampoules.)

The total volume to be infused is 1000 ml of dextrose 5% plus 36.75 ml acetylcysteine = 1036.75 ml.

This is to be infused over 16 hours.

So the infusion rate = 1036.75/16 ml per hour = 64.796875 ml/h. This can be rounded to 65 ml/h.

15.1   Calculate the volumes required for the following doses and concentrations:

(a) a dose of 200 mg of flucloxacillin, available in a preparation containing 250 mg in 5ml;

(b) an intravenous injection of 75 mg of metronidazole, available in a bag with concentration of 0.5% w/v;

(c) 0.5 mg of Drug A available as an intravenous preparation with concentration 250 micrograms/ml.

15.2   A child aged 10 years is admitted to hospital with a severe infection. On investigation it is found that the infection is sensitive to benzylpenicillin.

Benzylpenicillin is prescribed at a dose of 100 mg/kg daily and is administered in 4 equally divided doses by intravenous infusion.

On admission the child is weighed and found to be 30 kg.

(Continued)

HAVE A CHECK-UP

(Continued)

(a) What is the total daily dose required for this child?

(b) What is the dosage required for each single administration?

15.3 A patient is prescribed 1.5 g of Drug B as an intravenous injection. Available as stock are 750-mg vials of Drug B. A vial is reconstituted for injection using water to a total volume of 10 ml. How many millilitres will be administered to deliver the correct dose?

15.4 A patient requires an injection of 350 mg aminophylline. This drug is available in a concentration of 1% w/v. What volume should be injected?

15.5 A child aged 9 months requires a daily dose of Drug C, for which the recommended dosage is 1.5 mg/m². The child has a weight of 9.5 kg and a height of 74 cm. Calculate the dose required.

15.6 A dose of 1.5 g of potassium chloride is to be added to a litre of sodium chloride 0.9% solution. Available are 10-ml ampoules of potassium chloride 20% solution (w/v). What volume should be drawn up?

15.7 An adult patient is prescribed aciclovir 5 mg/kg three times daily by intravenous infusion. The patient weighs 70 kg. Aciclovir is available in vials containing 500 mg in 20 ml.

(a) What amount is required for each single dose?

(b) What volume is required to be administered for each single dose?

15.8 A child weighing 32 kg is prescribed metronidazole by intravenous infusion at a dose of 7.5 mg/kg every 8 hours.

Intravenous metronidazole is supplied in pre-prepared bags containing 100ml and a dosage of 5 mg per ml.

(a) What amount is required for each single dose?

(b) What is the volume required to administer the correct dose to the child?

15.9 An adult weighing 72 kg is prescribed gentamicin at a dose of 5 mg per kg once daily.

Available for intravenous injection are 2-ml vials containing 40 mg of gentamicin per ml.

(a) What is the correct dose of gentamicin in mg to be given each day?

(b) How many mls are required to administer a single dose?

(c) How many vials are required to deliver this dose?

15.10 Access the growth charts for boys 0–4 years on the RCPCH website.

Baby Ben, aged 12 weeks, is found to weigh 5.2 kg, to have a length of 58 cm and to have a head circumference of 39.0 cm.

(a) Approximately, what are the median values of weight, length and head circumference for boys of 12 weeks?

(b) Approximately, what are the ranges of values that lie within the 25th and 75th percentiles (centiles) for these three measurements for boys of 12 weeks?

(c) With respect to these three measurements, how does baby Ben compare with other children of this age?

15.11   Refer to the growth charts for boys 0–4 years on the RCPCH website, which include a weight-height to BMI conversion chart for children over 2 years.

William, aged 45 weeks, weighs 20.5 kg and has a height of 104 cm.

(a) Convert William's weight and height to approximate percentiles for boys of age 45 weeks.

(b) Use the weight-height to BMI conversion chart to determine the approximate percentile (centile) equivalence for William's body-mass index.

(c) Interpret the result obtained in (b).

15.12   A patient who weighs 80 kg is receiving an infusion of Drug D running at 10 micrograms/kg/min. A pharmacy-prepared bag contains 1 g in 500 ml. What is the correct rate at which the infusion pump should be set in ml per hour?

15.13   A patient is prescribed heparin to treat a deep vein thrombosis.

An initial loading dose of 5000 units is given by intravenous injection and this is to be followed by a continuous intravenous infusion of 18 units per kg per hour.

The patient weighs 75 kg and the infusion is made up of 25 000 units of heparin in 500 ml 5% dextrose.

(a) What is the rate in ml/hr at which the infusion pump will be set to deliver the correct dosage?

(b) How long will the whole infusion take?

15.14   Lucy, aged 10 years, has been prescribed intravenous metronidazole at a dose of 7.5 mg/kg every 8 hours. Metronidazole is available as a 100-ml infusion bag containing 5 mg/ml. Lucy is weighed and found to be 32.5 kg.

(a) What dosage is required every 8 hours for Lucy?

(b) What volume of the prepared infusion bag is required to be infused?

(c) The infusion is to be administered over 20 minutes. What rate should the infusion pump be set at to deliver the drug in the required time?

15.15   (a) An adult patient who weighs 80 kg is given an initial dose of 25 ng/kg of Drug E daily. What is the dose in micrograms for this patient?

(Continued)

(Continued)

   (b) Following review this dose is increased by 20%. What is the increased dose in micrograms?

15.16   Sugar-free oral drops of alfacalcidol are available in a concentration of 2 micrograms/ml. There are approximately 20 drops in 1 ml. How many nanograms are there approximately in one drop?

15.17   Jake, a 7-year-old boy with a cardiac abnormality, weighs 28 kg. He is prescribed 75% of normal maintenance fluids over 24 hours. Jake is receiving an infusion amounting to 16.7 ml/hour of fluid. He is also receiving other medication which amounts to a further 15 ml every six hours.

   (a) Use the formula given earlier in the chapter for Example 15.10 to calculate Jake's total fluid requirement over 24 hours.

   (b) How much fluid per hour, in addition to the infusion and other medication, should Jake be given?

15.18   Approximately how many millimoles of sodium are there in a 10-ml ampoule of sodium chloride 0.9%? The molecular mass of sodium chloride is 58.5 and the chemical formula is NaCl (Na = sodium, Cl = chlorine).

15.19   A volume of 30 mmol of potassium chloride is to be added to a 1-litre infusion. An ampoule contains 2 g of potassium chloride in 10 ml. What volume should be drawn up? (The molecular mass of potassium chloride is 74.5.)

15.20   1 gram of diamorphine powder displaces 6 ml of water. In what volume of water should 400 mg of diamorphine be reconstituted to produce a total volume of 20 ml?

ANSWERS TO CHECK-UPS

Chapter 1

1.1 (a) 2 thousands; (b) 2×10^3; (c) no tens.

1.2 (a) 2 hundredths; (b) 2×10^{-2}; (c) no thousandths.

1.3 The largest is 5.61 and the smallest is 5.016.

1.4 (a) 0.085

(b) 0.105.

1.5 (a) 1×10^7 is 1 followed 7 zeros; a million is 1 followed by 6 zeros. 1×10^7 is the larger.

(b) 1×10^{-7} is 1 divided by ten 7 times; a millionth is 1 divided by ten 6 times. 1×10^{-7} is the smaller.

1.6 (a) 0.01 or 0.010 (b) About 2 miles down the road to your right!

1.7 A is 2.86; B is 3.01; C is about 3.095.

1.8 The missing labels are 0.29, 0.30, 0.31 and 0.32.

1.9 (a) 0.275 is 275 thousandths; (b) 25.6 is 256 tenths; (c) 12.5 = 12.50, which is 1250 hundredths; (d) 1.05 = 1.050, which is 1050 thousandths.

Chapter 2

We suggest ways of doing these additions and subtractions, but you may well have different but equally effective ways of doing them.

2.1 (a) 8 + 7 = 15, so 800 + 700 = 1500; total cost = £1500. (b) The difference between 15 and 8 is 7; so the difference between £15 000 and £8000 is £7000.

2.2 (a) 72 (b) 35 (c) 100 (d) 156 (e) 158 (f) 37 (g) 83 (h) 8 (i) 96 (j) 8

2.3 The number lines might be completed as shown below, giving (a) 127 + 39 = 166, (b) 217 − 148 = 69.

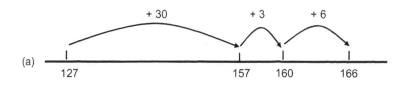

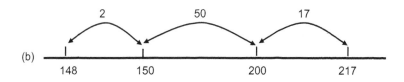

2.4 (a) 538 + 294 = (500 + 30 + 8) + (200 + 90 + 4) = 700 + 120 + 12 = 832

(b) 423 + 98 = 423 + 100 − 2 = 523 − 2 = 521

(c) 394 + 307 = 394 + 6 + 301 = 400 + 301 = 701

(d) 297 + 304 = 300 − 3 + 300 + 4 = 600 + 4 − 3 = 601

2.5 (a) 1000 − 450 = 550, so 1000 − 448 = 552

(b) 720 − 520 = 200, so 719 − 520 = 199

(c) 725 − 487 = 3 + 10 + 200 + 25 = 238

(d) 7020 − 6994 = 7026 − 7000 = 26

(e) 5000 − 17 = 5000 − 20 + 3 = 4980 + 3 = 4983

2.6 Check that: (a) 552 + 448 = 1000; (b) 199 + 520 = 719; (c) 238 + 487 = 725; (d) 26 + 6994 = 7020; (e) 4983 + 17 = 5000.

2.7 (a) 396 + 172 should equal 568 (b) 405 − 144 should equal 261

(c) this is correct   (d) 3003 − 749 should equal 2254

2.8 (a) 2121 (b) 1645 (c) 2229

(d) 2015 (e) 2312 (f) 2015

(g) 2395 (h) 2065

The fluid balance is 2395 – 2065 = 330 (positive).

Chapter 3

We suggest ways of doing the multiplications and divisions required here, but you may well have different but equally effective ways of doing them.

3.1 The numbers in the top row are multiples of 6: 36, 42, 48, 54.

The next row, multiples of 7: 42, 49, 56, 63.

Then multiples of 8: 48, 56, 64, 72.

And in the bottom row, multiples of 9: 54, 63, 72, 81.

3.2 (a) $7 \times 1 = 7$, $7 \times 2 = 14$, $7 \times 3 = 21$, $7 \times 4 = 28$, $7 \times 5 = 35$, $7 \times 6 = 42$, $7 \times 7 = 49$, $7 \times 8 = 56$, $7 \times 9 = 63$, $7 \times 10 = 70$.

(b) Every 8 hours is 3 times a day: so we use $7 \times 3 = 21$.

3.3 (a) $12 \times 5 = 6 \times 2 \times 5 = 6 \times 10 = 60$; (b) $50 \times 8 = 50 \times 2 \times 4 = 100 \times 4 = 400$; (c) $25 \times 12 = 25 \times 4 \times 3 = 100 \times 3 = 300$; (d) $15 \times 30 = (10 \times 30) + (5 \times 30) = 300 + 150 = 450$; (e) $99 \times 7 = (100 \times 7) - (1 \times 7) = 700 - 7 = 693$.

3.4 (a) $600 \div 5$ (double both numbers) $= 1200 \div 10 = 120$; (b) $250 \div 25 = 10$ (because $25 \times 10 = 250$); (c) $120 \div 24$ (divide both by 12) $= 10 \div 2 = 5$; (d) $96 \div 3 = (90 \div 3) + (6 \div 3) = 30 + 2 = 32$; (e) $360 \div 90$ (divide both numbers by 10) $= 36 \div 9 = 4$ (because we know $4 \times 9 = 36$).

3.5 (a) $100 \div 25 = 4$ capsules; (b) $175 \div 25 = (100 + 75) \div 25 = (100 \div 25) + (75 \div 25) = 4 + 3 = 7$ capsules.

3.6 $5037 \div 69 = 73$ and $5037 \div 73 = 69$.

3.7 (a) $28 \times 1 = 28$, $28 \times 2 = 56$, $28 \times 3 = 84$, $28 \times 4 = 112$, $28 \times 5 = 140$, $28 \times 6 = 168$, $28 \times 7 = 196$, $28 \times 8 = 224$, $28 \times 9 = 252$, $28 \times 10 = 280$.

(b) $28 \times 5 = 140$, which tells us that 5 packets are needed for 140 tablets.

3.8   (a) 100 ÷ 28 = 3 remainder 16; (b) for 100 tablets 3 packs of 28 plus 16 additional tablets would be required.

3.9   (a) 2 tablets 4 times a day for 14 days = 2 × 4 × 14 = 112 tablets; (b) 4 packs.

3.10 83 × 12 = (83 × 10) + (83 × 2) = 830 + 166 = 996 millilitres.

3.11 0.009 × 100 = 0.9 (grams)

3.12 1.8 ÷ 100 = 0.018 (grams)

3.13 75 × 24 = 1800 (millilitres)

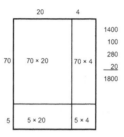

3.14 We check to see if 25 × 16 is equal to 450. In fact, 25 × 16 = 25 × 4 × 4 = 100 × 4 = 400. So the division is incorrect. The correct result is 450 ÷ 25 = 18.

3.15 (a) and (d) are correct. In (b) the first step of 11 divided by 5 gives 2 carry 1; what is recorded here is 1 carry 2. The correct answer should be 225. In (c) the decimal point above the line must be positioned above the decimal point below the line; the correct answer is 24.25

Chapter 4

4.1   2.094 m (Note: this is 2 m + 0 dm + 9 cm + 4 mm)

4.2   (a) Multiply by 1000, so 1.4 m = 1400 mm

      (b) Divide by 100, so 105 cm = 1.05 m

      (c) Multiply by 10, so 0.7 cm = 7 mm

      (d) Divide by 1000, so 75 mm = 0.075 m

4.3   Expressing all the lengths in millimetres, they are in the order given: 495 mm, 459 mm, 4059 mm, 500 mm. Of these (a) the longest is 4059 mm, and (b) the shortest is 459 mm (0.459 m).

4.4   Halfway between 46 cm and 47 cm is 46.5 cm, which is 465 mm.

4.5   The height indicated is 103.6 cm, which is 1.036 m.

4.6   The height of 1.39 m is 139 cm. When increased by 1 cm this becomes 140 cm. The new height is 1.40 m.

Chapter 5

5.1   You may be able to argue for different answers, but we think these are reasonable!

A wall-mounted hand sanitizer dispenser	0.8 litres (800 ml)
A vial of the antibiotic gentamicin	2 ml
A small bottle of water	250 ml
A syringe for a blood sample sufficient for a range of tests	20 ml
A hospital cleaner's bucket	5.7 litres
A small glass of wine (5 glasses per bottle)	150 ml

5.2   (a) 1.25 litres = 1250 ml; (b) 1400 ml = 1.400 litres (or 1.4 litres); (c) 0.05 litres = 50 ml; (d) 6 ml = 0.006 litres.

5.3   By converting all the volumes to millilitres the list becomes: 500 ml, 525 ml, 65 ml, 530 ml, 99 ml. So, (a) the largest volume is the 530 ml (0.53 litres); and (b) the smallest volume is the 65 ml (0.065 litres).

5.4   A dose of 0.1 ml is smaller than 1 ml, so the 1-ml syringe would have to be used. The dose drawn would come only one tenth of the way along the scale marked on the syringe.

5.5   (a) In 8 hours at 20 ml each hour a total volume of 160 ml would be delivered; (b) this is 0.16 litres (or 0.160 litres).

5.6   (a) A volume of 0.6 litres is 600 millilitres. The volume to be delivered per hour is therefore 600 ÷ 5 = 120 ml. (b) 0.12 litres (or 0.120 litres).

5.7   (a) 250 ml + 375 ml + 400 ml + 180 ml + 245 ml = 1450 ml; (b) 1.45 litres (or 1.450 litres).

Chapter 6

6.1   (a) 1.25 mg = 1250 micrograms; (b) 7250 g = 7.250 kg (or 7.25 kg).

6.2.   By converting all the weights to milligrams the list becomes: 500 mg, 275 mg, 5 mg, 600 mg, 6 mg. So, (a) the largest dose is the 600 mg (0.6 g), and (b) the smallest dose is the 5 mg (5000 micrograms).

6.3   Think of the 1.5 g as 1500 mg. Then by mental calculation (halve 1500 and halve again) we get 1500 ÷ 4 = 375. So the dose of erythromycin every 6 hours is (a) 375 mg, or (b) 0.375 g.

6.4   We need both measurements in the same unit: so change the 4 g to 4000 mg. Now, divide 4000 by 50 (= 80). So, 80 doses of 50 mg of Drug A are required.

6.5   We need 70 amounts of 5 mg of Drug B. Multiply 5 by 70 (= 350). So the dosage is (a) 350 mg, or (b) 0.350 g (or 0.35 g).

Chapter 7

7.1   The result displayed on the calculator for 47.5 × 24 is 1140. This means the total volume delivered daily is (a) 1140 ml, or (b) 1.140 litres. The result 1140 looks reasonable. An approximation would be 50 × 24, which we can do mentally, getting the result 1200 (50 × 24 = 100 × 12). So for 47.5 × 24 we would expect an answer a bit less than 1200.

7.2   Our calculator result for 47.5 ÷ 60 was 0.79166667, which means a drip rate of about 0.79 ml per minute. To check this by using inverse operations we would multiply the calculator result by 60. When we did this, on our calculator we got an answer that was just a tiny bit greater than the 47.5 we were expecting: 47.5000002. We recognized this as an insignificant rounding error. It was close enough to 47.5 for us to be confident we had the right answer.

7.3   The calculator answer for 29 × 7.5 is 217.5, which is interpreted as a dose of (a) 217.5 mg, or (b) 0.2175 g. A way of checking that the answer 217.5 is reasonable would be to note that 29 × 7.5 is approximately 30 × 7, which is 210. So 217.5 looks about the right magnitude.

7.4   To calculate 12 × 4 + 16 × 2 on a basic calculator without writing down any intermediate results you could follow this sequence:

- clear the memory by pressing *MC*
- enter '12 × 4 =' followed by *M+* to add this result to the memory
- enter '16 × 2 =' followed by *M+* to add this result to the memory
- press *MR* to display the result.

This example is included for illustrative purposes. In practice we would expect you just to write down 48 + 32 and find the total 80 mentally.

7.5   (a) On a scientific calculator you could enter the expression exactly as it is: '7 × 6 + 7 × 5 + 7 × 4 + 7 × 3 + 7 × 2 + 7 =', getting the result 147. The calculator automatically does each multiplication before adding the result to the current total. The first time Paul did this calculation on his calculator he got the result 980; professional common sense told him that 980 tablets could not possibly be right, so he did it again and got the correct result second time round!

(b) On a basic calculator, you could follow this sequence:

- clear the memory by pressing MC
- enter '7 × 6 =' followed by M+ to add this result to the memory
- enter '7 × 5 =' followed by M+ to add this result to the memory
- and so on for each of '7 × 4 =', '7 × 3 =', '7 × 2 =', adding each result to the memory by pressing M+
- enter 7 followed by M+
- press MR to display the result.

This example is included for illustrative purposes. In practice we would expect you just to write down 42 + 35 + 28 + 21 + 14 + 7 and find the total 147 mentally.

Chapter 8

8.1   (a) 7.5 ml, (b) 15.5 ml, (c) 3.5 ml

8.2   (a) 27 mg, (b) 27.1 mg, (c) 27.10 mg (d) 27.1 mg.

Part (c) is tricky, so well done if you got this right! The diagram below shows that 27.096667 lies between 27.09 and 27.10, and that it is closer to 27.10.

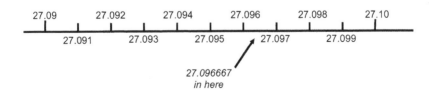

8.3 (a) 0.1 g (Note that 0.08764 lies between 0.0 and 0.1, and is closer to 0.1)

(b) 0.09 g, (c) 0.088 g, (d) 0.0876 g.

8.4   Using a calculator, 375 ÷ 24 = 15.625, so rounded to the nearest millilitre the required volume is 16 ml.

8.5   Using a calculator, 1031.75 ÷ 16 = 64.484375, so rounded to the nearest millilitre the infusion rate to be set is 64 ml per hour.

8.6   Using a calculator, 1031.75 ÷ 64 = 16.1210938, or about 16.12 hours. That is about 7 minutes over the 16 hours. This is a rounding error. Because the volume to be infused per hour was rounded down (to 64 from 64.484375) it will take longer to complete the infusion. This is not significant in relation to the well-being of the patient.

Here's an interesting observation. If in question 8.5 the infusion rate had been set to one decimal place (or 3 significant digits) it would have been 64.5 ml per hour. Using this rate we can calculate the time taken for the infusion to be 1031.75 ÷ 64.5 = 15.996124 hours. This is actually only 14 seconds short of the required 16 hours for the infusion. So in this case rounding to one additional digit has made a big difference to the consequent rounding error: reducing it from 7 minutes over the16 hours to 14 seconds under.

Chapter 9

9.1   The completed grid is shown below. The number in the cell underneath the 0.7, for example, may be found by calculating 0.7 – 0.07; writing this as 0.70 – 0.07 leads to the result, 0.63 (compare 70 – 7 = 63). This number may also be found by calculating 0.23 + 0.4, which is 0.23 + 0.40.

Add 0.4

0.3	0.7	1.1	1.5	1.9
0.23	0.63	1.03	1.43	1.83
0.16	0.56	0.96	1.36	1.76
0.09	0.49	0.89	1.29	1.69
0.02	0.42	0.82	1.22	1.62

Subtract 0.07

9.2   The completed multiplication grid is shown below. To find the missing number in the column headings, use the fact that when this number is multiplied by 5 the result is 2.5. So the missing number is 2.5 ÷ 5 = 0.5. To find the missing number in the row headings, use the fact that when this number is multiplied by 0.8 the result is 1.6. So the missing number is 1.6 ÷ 0.8 (which equals 16 ÷ 8).

×	0.02	0.05	0.4	0.5	0.8
5	0.1	0.25	2	2.5	4
2	0.04	0.1	0.8	1	1.6
0.5	0.01	0.025	0.2	0.25	0.4
0.2	0.004	0.01	0.08	0.1	0.16
0.1	0.002	0.005	0.04	0.05	0.08

9.3 (a) 1 ml   (b) 0.5 mg   (c) 3 g (d) 0.25 mg

9.4 (a) 2 micrograms   (b) 1 g (d) 5 mg   (d) 0.5 litres

9.5 To find 20 × 0.2, first transform it in your mind to 20 × 2 = 40, then put back the one digit after the decimal point, to give the result 4.0. The dosage of GTN contained in 20 ml is 4.0 mg (or 4 mg).

Or, using factors: 20 × 0.2 = 2 × 10 × 0.2 = 2 × 2 = 4.

9.6 To find 2.5 × 72, first transform it in your mind to 25 × 72. Get the answer to this by an appropriate method (25 × 72 = 1800), then put back the one digit after the decimal point, to give the result 180.0.

Or, using factors: 2.5 × 72 = 2.5 × 4 × 18 = 10 × 18 = 180.

For this patient the infusion rate is therefore 180 micrograms per minute.

9.7 To find 20 × 12.5, first calculate 20 × 125 (= 2500), then put back the one digit after the decimal point, to give the result 250.0. The total amount of dobutamine in the ampoule is 250 mg.

Or, using factors: 20 × 12.5 = 10 × 2 × 12.5 = 10 × 25 = 250.

9.8 The calculation required is 20 ÷ 0.4. Multiply both numbers by 10 and this becomes 200 ÷ 4, giving the answer 50. So 50 doses are required.

9.9 The calculation required is 2 ÷ 0.04. Multiply both numbers by 100 and this becomes 200 ÷ 4, the same calculation as in question 9.8. So 50 doses are again required.

9.10 (a) This approximates to 0.03 × 8 = 0.24. The result (0.26) looks reasonable.

(b) This approximates to 20 × 0.08 = 1.60. The result (17.85) clearly has the decimal point in the wrong place.

(c) This approximates to 13 ÷ 0.05. Multiplying both numbers in this division by 100 gives 1300 ÷ 5, which is 260. The result (263) looks reasonable.

(d) This approximates to 0.09 ÷ 0.3. Multiplying both numbers in this division by 10 it becomes 0.9 ÷ 3, which equals 0.3. The result (0.00304) looks seriously wrong!

Chapter 10

10.1   The average birth weight of a baby born in Britain today is 7 lb 4 oz, but weight can vary widely, between about 5 lb 8 oz and 11 lb, with girls tending to be around 11 oz lighter than boys.

10.2   The average length of newborn babies in the UK is around 46 to 56 cm. They should normally grow about 2.5 to 3.8 cm in length during the first month.

10.3   (a) 2 metres (= 6 ft 6 ins) (b) 2 pints (= 1.14 litres) (c) 6 inches (= 15.2 cm) (d) 10 stone (= 63.5 kg) (e) 250 g (half a pound is about 227 g)

10.4   This is the result of rounding errors. To a higher level of accuracy 2.0 kg is 70.548 ounces (which is rounded up to 71 oz in the table in Figure 10.3). When doubled, this would give a weight of 4.0 kg as 141.096 ounces (which is rounded down in the table to 141 oz).

10.5   The weights in pounds and ounces, row by row, are as follows:

4 lb 7 oz, 4 lb 10 oz, 4 lb 14 oz, 5 lb 1 oz, 5 lb 5 oz

5 lb 8 oz, 5 lb 12 oz, 5 lb 15 oz, 6 lb 3 oz, 6 lb 6 oz

6 lb 10 oz, 6 lb, 13 oz, 7 lb 1 oz, 7 lb 4 oz, 7 lb 8 oz

7 lb 11 oz, 7 lb 15 oz, 8 lb 3 oz, 8 lb 6 oz, 8 lb 10 oz

8 lb 13 oz, 9 lb 1 oz, 9 lb 4 oz, 9 lb 8 oz, 9 lb 11oz

9 lb 15 oz, 10 lb 2 oz, 10 lb 6 oz, 10 lb 9 oz, 10 lb 13 oz

Chapter 11

11.1   (a) The fraction used is $^{12}/_{20}$, which in its simplest form cancels down to $^{3}/_{5}$ (dividing top and bottom by 4). (b) The fraction of the stock remaining is $^{2}/_{5}$.

11.2   Each beaker would contain $^{3}/_{18}$ of a litre. Cancelling 3, this simplifies to $^{1}/_{6}$ of a litre.

11.3 (a) The secretary's rise is $^7/_{10}$ of the nurse's rise. (b) The ratio of the secretary's rise to the nurse's rise is 7:10.

11.4 $6:9 = 2:3 = 18:27 = 600:900 = 1:1.5$ (you can get this by halving the numbers in the ratio 2:3)

11.5 (a) The ratio 5:4 is $1:^4/_5$. This is found by dividing both numbers by 5. This is written in decimal form as 1:0.8. (b) The ratio 5:4 is $^5/_4:1$. This is found by dividing both numbers by 4. This is written in decimal form as 1.25:1.

11.6 (a) Doubling both top and bottom numbers gives $^{22.5}/_{60} = ^{45}/_{120}$. To get this in its simplest form, cancel 15, giving $^3/_8$. (b) The rate is 0.375 ml per minute.

11.7 (a) $^{25}/_4 = 6^1/_4$ (b) The dose is 6.25 mg.

11.8 Example 11.2: each dose is 0.625 g.

Example 11.4: each dose is 0.75 g.

Example 11.9: (a) 12.5 ml; (b) 3.75 g.

11.9 (a) 0.5 °C   (b) 0.25 litres   (c) 0.9 cm   (d) 0.07 m (e) 0.875 g

(f) 0.4 litres (g) 0.36 mg   (h) 0.06 kg (i) 2.25 ml (j) 1.75 hours

11.10 As a mixed number $^{13}/_3$ is $4^1/_3$, which in decimal form is 4.33 (to 3 significant digits)

11.11 To find $^1/_6$ as a decimal, divide 1 by 6 to get 0.1666666..., which is 0.167 to 3 significant digits.

To find $^2/_6$ as a decimal, we can cancel 2 to get $^1/_3$, which we know is 0.333.

To find $^3/_6$ as a decimal, we can cancel 3 to get $^1/_2$, which we know is 0.5.

To find $^4/_6$ as a decimal, we can cancel 2 to get $^2/_3$, which we know is 0.667.

To find $^5/_6$ as a decimal, subtract the decimal equivalent of $^1/_6$ from 1. This gives us $1 - 0.167 \approx 0.833$.

11.12 Doubling top and bottom, $^{2.5}/_{30} \approx ^5/_{60}$. From 11.11 we know that $^5/_6$ is 0.833; $^5/_{60}$ will be a tenth of this. So, $^5/_{60} = 0.0833$. Hence the concentration is 0.0833 mg per ml (which is 83.3 micrograms per ml).

11.13 The value of $^{50}/_6$ will be 10 times the value of $^5/_6$ (0.833) which gives the dose to be 8.33 mg. Alternatively, we could cancel 2 in

$^{50}/_6$ to get $^{25}/_3$, which as a mixed number is $8^1/_3$. This can then be written as a decimal, again giving the dose as 8.33 mg.

11.14 (a) 0.208 litres (b) 0.283 hours (c) 0.024 kg

11.15 (a) 2 and $^2/_5$ hours (b) 2 hours and 24 minutes

11.16 (a) $^9/_{10}$ of a litre

(b) $^8/_{100}$ of a gram, which simplifies to $^2/_{25}$ of a gram

(c) $^{125}/_{1000}$ of a metre, which cancels down to $^1/_8$ of a metre

(d) $3^{25}/_{100}$ mg, which cancels down to $3^1/_4$ mg

11.17 (a) $7^1/_2 = 7.5$, so the fraction delivered so far is $^{7.5}/_{12}$. To simplify this double both numbers to get $^{15}/_{24}$. Then cancel 3 to get $^5/_8$.

(b) We have to calculate $^5/_8$ of 1000 ml. The calculation required is $1000 \div 8 \times 5$, which equals 625. So the volume delivered is 625 ml.

11.18 (a) $^3/_5$ of 40 = 24 tablets (one fifth of 40 is 8, then multiply by 3)

(b) $^7/_8$ of 600 ml = 525 (one eighth of 600 is 75, then multiply by 7)

(c) $^5/_6$ of 120 mg = 100 mg (one sixth of 120 mg is 20 mg, then multiply by 5)

Chapter 12

12.1 The completed arrays are shown below, with arrows indicating what seem to us the easiest (but not the only) ways to get the answers: (a) 360 × 3 = 1080 g; (b) 7 × 90 = 630 g; (c) 550/90 = 55/9 = 6.11 ... this is rounded down to 6 people.

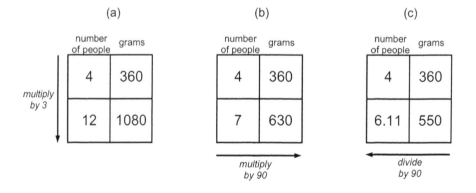

12.2 (a) £1.50 × 4.5 = £6.75   (b) 56/7 = 8, so £8 per metre

      (c) 15/45 = $^1/_3$ of an hour = 20 minutes

12.3 (a) 33 beats in 15 seconds   (b) 48 beats per minute

12.4 (a) The information given tells us that 10 ml contains
          750 mg. We need to calculate the volume corresponding to
          1500 mg. Answer: 20 ml. Below we show one way of
          finding the 20 ml.

      (b) The information given tells us that 10 ml contains 500 mg of
          Drug K. We need to calculate the dose of Drug K corresponding
          to 25 ml. Answer: 1250 mg (= 1.25 g). Below we show one way
          of finding the 1250 mg.

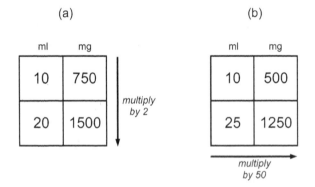

12.5 The answers are: (a) 9 ml; (b) 12.5 ml; (c) 37.5 ml; (d) 3.5 ml.

      The diagrams that follow show how these might be calculated.

      (a) We get from 100 to 5 by dividing by 20, so 180 is divided by
          20: 180/20 = 18/2 = 9 ml.

      (b) We get from 10 to 5 by dividing by 2, so 25 is divided by 2:
          25/2 = 12.5 ml.

      (c) First 1.5 g is written as 1500 mg. We get from 200 to 5 by
          dividing by 40, so 1500 is divided by 40: 1500/40 = 150/4 =
          75/2 = 37.5 ml.

      (d) We get from 40 to 4 by dividing by 10, so 35 is divided by 10:
          35/10 = 3.5 ml.

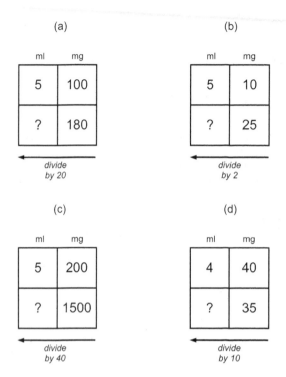

12.6 (a) 20 mg/ml (b) 2 mg/ml (c) 40 mg/ml (d) 10 mg/ml

12.7 (a) The number of units in a 10-ml vial with concentration 100 units/ml is 10 × 100 = 1000 units.

(b) We are told that there are 100 units of the drug in 1 ml. We must find the volume for 35 units. Using the model provided in Example 12.5(a) and (b), earlier in the chapter, we must divide 35 by the concentration. So the volume required is 35/100 = 0.35 ml.

12.8 (a) The dosage in a 50-ml vial with concentration 5 mg/ml is 50 × 5 = 250 mg.

(b) We have 5 mg in 1 ml. We need the volume for 125 mg, which is 25 times 5 mg, so we require 25 ml. We observe that this is half a 50-ml vial required for the dose of 125 mg, which is consistent with the fact that a vial contains 250 mg.

12.9 (a) The total daily dose is 100 × 30 mg = 3000 mg (or 3 g). (b) The 6-hourly dose is 3000/4 = 1500/2 = 750 mg.

12.10 (a) 250 × 4.0 = 1000 mg. (b) 1000/3 = 333 mg (to the nearest milligram).

12.11 The dose required is 1.5 × 0.6 = 0.9 mg.

12.12

Fluid	Volume infused	Time	Infusion rate
Dextrose 5%	1000 ml	8 hours	125 ml/h
Dextrose 5%	500 ml	4 hours	125 ml/h
Sodium chloride 0.9%	1000 ml	6 hours	167 ml/h
Sodium chloride 0.9%	1000 ml	12 hours	83 ml/h
Sodium chloride 0.9%	500 ml	6 hours	83 ml/h
Metronidazole 5 mg/ml	100 ml	1 hour	100 ml/h
Dextrose 5%	500 ml	4 hours	125 ml/h
Hartmann's solution	500 ml	3 hours	167 ml/h

12.13 Since 15 minutes is $1/4$ of an hour, the volume per hour will be 4 times the volume in 15 minutes. Hence the infusion rate is 30 × 4 = 120 ml/h.

12.14 (a) Infusion rate = 100 ml per hour.

(b) Each millilitre in a standard giving set is 20 drops. So 100 ml per hour is 100 × 20 = 2000 drops per hour = 2000/60 drops per minute. This can be cancelled down to 100/3 = 33 drops per minute (rounded to the nearest whole number).

12.15 (a) Infusion rate = 500/6 = 83.33... ml per hour, which is 83 ml/h to the nearest millilitre. Note: we will use 83.3 rather than 83 in subsequent calculations, to be cautious regarding rounding errors.

(b) Each millilitre in a standard giving set is 20 drops. So 83.3 ml per hour is 83.3 × 20 = 1666 drops per hour = 1666/60 drops per minute. This is probably best done on a calculator: 1666 ÷ 60 = 28 drops per minute (rounded to the nearest whole number).

12.16 (a) Infusion rate = 480/4 = 120 ml per hour.

(b) Each millilitre in a standard giving set for blood transfusion is 15 drops. So 120 ml per hour is 120 × 15 = 1800 drops per hour = 1800/60 drops per minute. This cancels down to 30 drops per minute.

12.17 A rate of 48 drops in 60 seconds is equivalent to 16 drops in 20 seconds (dividing by 3). If 18 drops are counted the rate is too high.

12.18 (a) The volume of iron dextran with a concentration of 50 mg/ml required to provide 800 mg is 800/50 = 16 ml.

(b) The total volume is 500 + 16 = 516 ml.

(c) To infuse 516 ml over 4 hours, the required rate is 516/4 = 129 ml/h.

Chapter 13

13.1   (a) 13%   (b) 91%

13.2   (a) 7 in 50 = 14 in 100 = 14%

(b) 150 per 1000 = 15 per 100 = 15%

(c) 24 out of 25 = 96 out of 100 = 96%

(d) 1 in 8 = $^1/_8$ = 12.5%

(e) 60 out of 90 = $^2/_3$ = 66.7%

(f) $^3/_5$ = 60%

(g) $^{73}/_{100}$ = 73%

(h) $^{68}/_{200}$ = $^{34}/_{100}$ = 34%

(i) $^1/_{30}$ = 0.0333 = 3.33%

(j) 0.01 in 100 = 0.01%

13.3 $^{72}/_{120}$ = $^6/_{10}$ (cancelling 12) = 60%

13.4   95 in 120 = 95/120 in 1 = 0.792 in 1 = 79.2 in 100 = 79.2%

13.5   (a) 0.2 g per 100 ml (b) 2 g per litre (c) 2 milligrams per ml

13.6   (a) 0.8 g per 100 ml (b) 8 g per litre (c) 8 milligrams per ml

13.7   This means that the supplier cannot guarantee that the product is 100% pure isopropyl alcohol. The 99.9% is 99.9 in 100, which is equivalent to 999 in 1000. The supplier guarantees the product meets the standard of at least 999 ml of isopropyl alcohol in 1000 ml.

13.8   (a) The 5% w/w means 5 mg of active ingredients in 100 mg of cream. (b) This is equivalent to 50 mg per 1000 mg, or 50 mg per gram.

13.9   Aciclovir 5% w/w contains 5 g of aciclovir per 100 g of cream. Dividing by 50, this is equivalent to 0.1 g per 2 g of cream. The 2-gram tube therefore contains 0.1 g or 100 mg of aciclovir.

13.10   (a) 80% of 200 mg = 0.8 × 200 mg = 160 mg

(b) 75% of 500 ml = $^3/_4$ of 500 ml = 375 ml

(c) 90% of 50 ml = $^9/_{10}$ of 50 ml = 45 ml

13.11   The reduced daily dosage is 70% of 120 mg = 0.7 × 120 mg = 84 mg

13.12   A can be any number! For example, 37% of 20 = 7.4 and 20% of
37 = 7.4.

It is always the case that A% of B = B% of A. This trick can sometimes be quite useful. For example, to calculate 36% of 25 mg
we could instead find 25% of 36 mg, which is much easier to do
because it's just a quarter of 36 mg.

13.13   14% v/v gives 14 ml in 100 ml = 7 ml in 50 ml = 21 ml in 150 ml.
A volume of 10 ml of alcohol is a 'unit' of alcohol, so this glass
contains just over 2 units.

13.14   2% w/v is 2 g in 100 ml. The dosage in a 20-ml ampoule will
therefore be $^1/_5$ of 2 g, which is 0.4 g, or 400 mg.

13.15   The normal total daily dose of Drug K for a patient weighing
60 kg is 60 × 100 mg = 6000 mg (6 g). The reduced dosage is
75% of this, which is 4500 mg, or 4.5 g.

13.16   500 is reduced by 75. So we need 75 as percentage of 500.
Dividing by 5, 75 in 500 is equal to 15 in 100, or 15%. There is a
15% reduction.

13.17   The price increases from £3.75 by 30p. Writing the £3.75 in
pence (375p), then we need to express 30 as a percentage of
375. As a fraction $^{30}/_{375}$ cancels down to $^2/_{25}$, which is equivalent
to $^8/_{100}$, or 8%. Alternatively, divide 30 by 375 on a calculator to
get the result as a decimal, 0.08, which is also equivalent to 8%.

13.18   The weight loss is 0.5 kg. Dividing this by the birth weight, using
a calculator: 0.5/3.7 = 0.135 = 13.5%.

13.19   (a) The patient's weight loss is 20% of his normal 80 kg, which
equals 16 kg. So on discharge he weighed 64 kg.

(b) The gain of 20% of the weight on discharge of 64 kg is a gain
of 12.8 kg. So his weight now is 64 + 12.8 = 76.8 kg.

Note that losing 20% and then gaining 20% does not get you
back to where you were! This is because the second 20% is 20%
of the reduced weight, which is less than 20% of the original
weight.

Chapter 14

14.1 $n = 11$ (11 is the only whole number that lies between 10 and 15,
and also lies between 7 and 12)

14.2 $d = (15 × 500)/240 = 7500/240 = 750/24 = 250/8 = 125/4 = 31.25$.

The drop rate would therefore be set at 31 drops per minute.

14.3 $T_C = [5(100 - 32)]/9 = (5 \times 68)/9 = 340/9 = 37.8$. The temperature is 37.8 °C to 3 significant digits.

14.4   (a) The values in order are: 3, 9.49, 30, 94.9, 300, 949.

   (b) Using the pattern in (a), the next two values in this sequence will be $\sqrt{9\,000\,000} = 3000$ and $\sqrt{90\,000\,000} = 9490$.

14.5   (a) The line joining 146 cm on the height scale to 48 kg on the weight scale intersects the BSA scale at 1.39. So an estimate for the BSA of this woman is 1.39 m². (b) Using the formula, BSA $= \sqrt{[(146 \times 48)/3600]} = \sqrt{1.947} = 1.40$ (to 3 significant digits), which is very close to the reading in (a).

14.6   The boy's height must first be converted to 93 cm. Then the BSA $= \sqrt{[(93 \times 16.5)/3600]} = 0.6529$ m². The weekly dosage is therefore $30 \times 0.6529 = 19.6$ mg (to one decimal place).

14.7   (a) Overweight; (b) underweight; (c) healthy weight.

14.8   Remember to convert the height to metres. Then BMI $= 90/(1.71^2) = 31$ (to the nearest whole number). This is not a healthy weight for this man; he is very overweight.

14.9   The height and weight must be converted to metres and kilograms. See Chapter 10. The height of 4 feet 8 inches $=$ 56 inches $= 56 \times 2.54$ cm $= 142$ cm $= 1.42$ m. The weight 10 stone 1 pound $= 141$ lb $= 141/2.2$ kg $= 64.1$ kg. So the woman's BMI is $64.1/(1.42^2) = 64.1/2.02 = 31.7 = 32$ to the nearest whole number.

14.10 (a) The 91st percentile weight for boys aged 3 weeks is about 4.8 kg. This means that the heaviest 9% of boys of this age weigh 4.8 kg or more.

   (b) Harry's weight is well below the 9th percentile. This means he is very underweight compared to boys of his age; his weight puts him in the bottom 9% for weight.

   (c) The median weight for boys aged 6 weeks is the 50th percentile, which is about 4.9 kg.

14.11 $(25 + 26 + 28 + 29 + 26 + 24 + 23)/7 = 181/7 = 25.9$ °C (to one decimal place).

14.12 (a) 1 mol of potassium chloride is 74.5 g.

   (b) 35 mmol is 0.035 mol. Using the result in (a), 0.035 mol of potassium chloride is 74.5 g x 0.035 = 2.6075 g. So, 35 mmol is 2.6075 g.

   (c) Sodium chloride 0.9% is a concentration of 0.9 g per 100 ml, or 9 g per litre. So we need to find how many millimoles are equivalent to 9 g. From the molecular mass, we know that 1 mole (1000 mmol) of sodium chloride is 58.5 g. So, 1 g is equivalent to 1000/58.5 mmol = 17.09 mmol. Hence, 9 g is equivalent to 17.09 × 9 = 154 mmol (to 3 significant digits). The concentration is 154 mmol per litre.

(d) Because the molecular mass is 58.5, 1 mol per litre would be 58.5 g per litre.This is equivalent to 5.85 g per 100 ml. So the concentration would be 5.85% (w/v).

(e) The molecular mass of sodium phosphate is 358. So 1 mol weighs 358 g. Hence 0.5 mol is equivalent to half this, which is 179 g. The concentration is therefore 179 g/litre, which is 17.9 g per 100 ml, or 17.9% w/v.

Chapter 15

15.1 (a) 250 mg in 5 ml is equivalent to 50 mg in 1 ml. So, for 200 mg a volume of 4 ml is required. (b) The concentration is 0.5 g per 100 ml. This is equivalent to 500 mg per 100 ml, or 5 mg/ml. For 75 mg, we require 75/5 = 15 ml. (c) The concentration is 250 micrograms/ml. We require 0.5 mg, which is 500 micrograms. The volume required is therefore 2 ml.

15.2 (a) Total dose = 30 × 100 mg = 3000 mg = 3 g. (b) Each single dose = 3000/4 = 750 mg (or 0.75 g).

15.3 The patient requires 1.5 g = 1500 mg of Drug B. One vial contains 750 mg, so 2 vials are used. The volume to be administered is therefore two lots of 10 ml, which equals 20 ml.

15.4 The concentration is 1 g per 100 ml, which is 1000 mg per 100 ml, which is equivalent to 10 mg/ml. For 350 mg, a volume of 35 ml is required.

15.5 An estimate for the child's BSA is $\sqrt{(74 \times 9.5/3600)}$ = 0.442 m². The dose required is 1.5 × 0.442 mg = 0.66 mg (rounded to 2 decimal places).

15.6 A 20% w/v concentration is 20 g per 100 ml. For 1 g we require 100/20 ml = 5 ml. Then for 1.5 g we need 1.5 × 5 = 7.5 ml; so the volume to be drawn up is 7.5 ml.

15.7 (a) Each dose is 70 × 5 mg = 350 mg.

(b) The concentration is 500 mg in 20 ml, which is 25 mg/ml. So the volume required is 350/25 = 14 ml.

15.8 (a) Each dose is 32 × 7.5 mg. Calculation: 32 × 7.5 = 16 × 15 = 8 × 30 = 240.

So the each single dose is 240 mg.

(b) The concentration is 5 mg/ml. So the volume required is 240/5 = 48 ml.

15.9   (a) For a patient weighing 72 kg the dose required is 72 × 5 mg = 360 mg.

(b) The concentration is 40 mg/ml, so the volume required for a single dose is 360/40 = 9 ml.

(c) Since each vial contains 2 ml, a total of 5 vials will be required to supply 9 ml ($4^1/_2$ vials are used).

15.10 (a) The median values (50th percentiles) are approximately: 5.7 kg for weight; 61 cm for length; and 40 cm for head circumference.

(b) The range of values from the 25th to 75th percentiles are approximately: 5.6 kg to 6.2 kg for weight; 59 cm to 62 cm for height; 39.5 cm to 41 cm for head circumference.

(c) All three of Ben's measurements come under the 25th percentile (but not lower than the 9th percentile). Compared to other boys of his age Ben is generally on the small side, but not exceptionally so.

15.11 (a) William is around the 98th percentile for weight and just under the 75th percentile for height.

(b) The point where the vertical line through the 75th percentile for height meets the horizontal line through the 98th percentile for weight lies between the diagonal lines representing the 98th and 99.6th percentiles for BMI.

(c) Children above the 98th percentile for BMI, like William, are categorized as clinically obese.

15.12 A rate of 10 microgram per kg per min for a patient of weight 80 kg is 80 x 10 = 800 micrograms per minute or 0.8 milligrams per minute. To convert this to milligrams per hour, multiply by 60: 0.8 × 60 = 8 × 6 = 48 mg/h. The bag contains 1 g in 500 ml, which is 1000 mg in 500 ml, which is equivalent to 2 mg/ml. So, for 48 mg we need 24 ml. The rate to be set is 24 ml/h.

15.13 The patient requires 18 units per kg per hour of heparin. A weight of 75 kg makes this 18 × 75 = 1350 units per hour.

We have three variables, units, volume and time, in proportion (compare Figure 15.2):

25 000 units	in 500 ml	in ? hours
1350 units	in ? ml	in 1 hour

(a) The missing numbers can be found using the principles of proportionality. The most obvious relationship to use is that 25 000 is divided by 50 to give 500. This gives the missing number in the second row to be 1350/50 = 27.

So the infusion rate is 27 ml per hour.

(b) If 27 ml is delivered in 1 hour, then 500 ml is delivered in 500/27 hours = 18.5 hours (approximately). This is the missing number in the top row above.

15.14   (a) For a weight of 32.5 kg the dose is 32.5 × 7.5 mg = 243.75 mg every 8 hours (using a calculator).

(b) The concentration in the infusion bag is 5 mg/ml, so the required volume is 243.75/5 ml = 48.75 ml.

(c) Note that 20 minutes is $^1/_3$ of an hour. So a rate of 48.75 ml in 20 minutes is equivalent to 48.75 × 3 ml per hour = 146.25 ml/h. Rounding this, the pump will be set to 146 ml/h.

15.15   (a) For a weight of 80 kg the initial dose is 80 × 25 ng = 2000 ng = 2 mg.

(b) Increasing 2 mg by 20% is increasing it by $^1/_5$ of 2 mg, which is 0.4 mg. So the increased dose is 2.4 mg.

15.16   A concentration of 2 micrograms in 1 millilitre is equivalent to 2000 nanograms in 1 millilitre. If 1 ml is approximately 20 drops, then each drop is approximately 2000/20 ng = 100 ng.

15.17   (a) Based on the formula given, the normal maintenance fluid requirement for a child weighing 28 kg is: (10 × 100) + (10 × 50) + (8 × 20) = 1660 ml over 24 hours. 75% of this is 1245 ml over 24 hours.

(b) This is equivalent to 1245/24 = 51.9 ml of fluid per hour. However the infusion is providing 16.7 ml per hour and other medication a further 15/6 ml per hour = 2.5 ml/h. So Jake's fluid requirement per hour in addition to these is 51.9 – (16.7 + 2.5) = 32.7 ml.

15.18   Sodium chloride 0.9% has a concentration of 0.9 g per 100 ml, which is 0.009 g per ml. So the amount of sodium chloride dissolved in a 10-ml ampoule is 10 × 0.009 = 0.09 g. We know that 58.5 g of sodium chloride is equivalent to 1000 mmol. So 0.09 g is equivalent to (0.09 × 1000)/58.5 = 1.54 mmol of sodium chloride, to three significant digits. Each molecule of NaCl contains one sodium ion. So in the solution the amount of sodium is also 1.54 mmol.

15.19   From the molecular mass we know that 74.5 g of potassium chloride is equivalent to 1 mol. The 30 mmol required is equal to 0.03 mol, which is equivalent therefore to 0.03 × 74.5 g = 2.235 g of potassium chloride. The concentration is 2 g in 10 ml, or 0.2 g/ml. So the volume required is 2.235/0.2 = 22.35/2 = 11.2 ml (to 1 decimal place).

15.20   If 1 g displaces 6 ml then 100 mg will displace 0.6 ml, and so 400 mg will displace 4 times this, which equals 2.4 ml. So the volume of water required to make up a total volume of 20 ml is 20 – 2.4 = 17.6 ml.

INDEX

accuracy, level of 11, 43, 85–6, 88–9, 91–93, 122, 139, 158
addition
    column method 24–5, 103–4
    mental strategies 15, 18–24, 101–3
    of multiples of ten, hundred, thousand 17
alcohol concentration 61, 175, 177
alcohol, unit of 61
algebra 188–9
algebraic operating system 76–8
approximation 59, 67, 80, 86, 112
area of rectangle 43–5
average
    birth weight 124
    BSA 190
    height 53
    median and mean 195–7
    speed 150
    weight 186, 195, 212
axis, axes (on a graph) 122–3, 125, 194, 213

blood glucose level 200
blood infusion 159–60
blood pressure 187
body length 50, 53, 120
body-mass index (BMI) 67, 92–3, 185–6, 192–4, 212–13
body surface area (BSA)
    in dosage calculation 81, 95–6, 107, 156–7, 205
    range of values 190
    using formula 184, 190-1
    using nomogram 191–2
brackets 32, 74–5, 77–8
bridging the gap (subtraction) 20–2, 26

brimful capacity 59
British Heart Foundation 192–3

calculators
    basic and scientific 74–7
    changing fractions into decimals 1 39–40, 151
    checking results 80–1
    find square root 75, 186, 190
    interpreting display 11
    memory keys 78–9
    percentage calculations 172, 178–9
    rounding results 88–96
    use in healthcare practice 79, 81, 202–19
cancelling fractions and ratios 130, 133–4, 138, 141, 167, 170, 206–7, 216
capacity 59
carrying one 25
centile 196
checking calculations 27, 34, 74, 80–1, 96, 112–13, 203
circumference of head 53, 196, 211–2
compensation (in addition and subtraction) 22–3
concentration
    expressed as a percentage 173–5
    in dosage calculations 153–6, 202–6
    moles or millimoles per litre 199–200, 213–14
    volume by volume 175
    weight by volume 173–5
conversion, imperial/metric units
    charts and tables 117, 119–22
    factors 124–5

conversion, imperial/metric units *cont.*
    reference items 123–4
    temperature 76–7, 125, 186–9
conversion between metric units
    length 53–5
    volume 61–2
    weight 68–71
cubed 3
cubic units 59

decimal numbers
    addition and subtraction 101–4
    changing to a fraction 140–1
    changing to a percentage 172
    divided by powers of ten 36–8
    division 43, 71, 109–13
    multiplication 104–9
    multiplied by powers of ten 36–8
    notation 7–12, 53
    recurring 139
    role of zero 6, 10–11
denominator 129, 133, 137, 139, 167,
    169–60
dependent/independent variables 188
digit 5
direct proportion 124, 149
displacement volume 214–15
division
    by number less than one 110
    by ten, hundred, thousand 37–8
    fundamental properties 31–4
    mental strategies 30–4, 42–3
    prerequisite skills 34–8
    remainder 43
    represented as a fraction 131–2
    short 45–6, 110–11
    with decimal numbers 43, 71, 109–13
dosage calculations 153–7, 202–6
drop rate calculations 159–61

equivalent
    divisions 42–3
    fractions 130, 132–4, 137–8, 167–71
    ratios 134–5, 151, 216
ET tube formulas 189
exchange, principle of 24–5

factors in calculations 41–2, 29–30, 108, 133,
    137, 151
fluid balance chart 23, 25, 27, 104

fluid requirements for children 209–11
formula (in algebra) 77, 184–6,
    188–93, 205
formula (chemical) 198, 213–14
fractions
    as divisions 131–2
    as proportions 129–31
    as ratios 132
    decimal equivalences 136–40
    equivalent 130, 132–4, 137–8, 167–71
    greater than one 136
    of a quantity 141–2
    percentage equivalences 169–72
friendlier numbers (in subtraction) 23–4
front-end approach 20

graph, graphical representation 121–5, 191,
    193–4
growth charts 195–6, 211–13

height 52–6, 84, 87, 92, 96, 116–20, 123
highest common factor 133

imperial units
    in healthcare practice 117
    metric equivalences 119–125
    of length 117–18
    of volume 119
inequality signs 187–8, 192
infusion pump 60–61, 94, 158, 208,
    215, 218
infusion rate calculations 88, 91, 94, 111,
    140, 157–61, 178, 199, 207–9, 217–9
infusion time 158, 208
inverse operations 33–4, 36–7, 42, 80–1, 134,
    173, 190

leading zero 8, 11, 62, 69
length
    abbreviations for units 51–3
    conversion of units 53–5
    imperial units 117–20, 123
    reference items 123
    units met in healthcare 51
limitations of measuring device 85

mass 67
mean of a set of data 196–7
measuring scale 6–7, 9–10, 50–2, 55–6, 59,
    87, 123–4

median value 195–6
medicine bottle 61
medicine spoon 59–60, 65, 67
microgram abbreviation 68
middle fifty percent 212
mixed number 134, 136, 140
mole, millimole, molar concentration
    197–200, 213–14
molecular mass 198–200, 213–14
Mosteller formula 191–2, 205
multiple 17–18, 30, 140
multiplication
    by multiples of ten, hundred,
        thousand 39
    by ten, hundred, thousand 36–8
    fundamental properties 31–4
    grid method 43–5
    mental strategies 30–4, 40–2
    with decimal numbers 104–9

negative powers of ten 7–8
neonate, new-born 53, 67, 91, 107, 118–123,
    126, 155–6
newton 68
nominal capacity 59
nomogram 184, 191–2, 205
number line
    empty 19, 21–23, 26, 104
    in rounding 88–9
    representing decimal numbers 9–10
    representing whole numbers 6–7
numeral 3–5, 7–8, 11, 59
numerator 129, 133, 139

Ordnance Survey map scale 135
origin (on a graph) 124–5

partitioning (in calculations) 20, 40, 44
per
    in drop rates 159–61
    in infusion rates 157–9
    kilogram of body weight 108, 152–3,
        204–6, 209–10, 216–19
    square metre of BSA 81, 107, 156–7,
        191, 205
    symbol for 154
    to relate two variables 152
percentage
    calculation 175–9
    concentration expressed as 173–5

percentage cont.
    increase and decrease 179–80
    meaning 167
    proportion expressed as 169–72
    related to decimals 172–3
    related to fractions 170
    use 169
percentile 186, 194–7, 211–13
place-holder, zero as 5, 8, 11, 37,
    62, 69
place value 3–12, 20, 24, 36–7, 53, 101
population 167, 186, 194–6, 212
powers of ten 3–8, 36, 198
precedence of operators 74, 77–8,
    186, 189
prefixes for measurement units 51–2, 59–60,
    67–8, 198
product 34–5, 40–2
proportion (fraction) 129–31
proportion problems 149–61, 203–4, 208,
    214, 216
proportional relationship 81, 124–5, 129,
    147–9, 152
pulse rate 152, 197

ratios
    equivalent 134–5
    in proportionality problems 147,
        149, 151
    one to something, something to one
        135–6
    represented as a fraction 132
recipe problems 161
rectangular array (for multiplication) 31–2,
    43–4
reference items 59, 67, 117, 123
rounding
    delayed 95, 218
    errors 80–1, 95–6, 139, 190, 218
    in healthcare contexts 77, 94, 140, 158,
        197, 218–19
    to a number of decimal places 91–2,
        191–2, 211, 213
    to check results 86, 96, 112–13
    to significant digits 86, 92–3, 111–12,
        118–20, 125, 139–40, 142, 172, 186,
        190, 207, 214
    to the nearest something 85–90, 107–8,
        121, 159–60
    up or down 90–91

Royal College of Paediatrics and Child
    Health (RCPCH) 195–6, 220–1

SI (Systeme Internationale) units
    51–2, 59
square of a number 3, 156, 190, 192
square root 186, 190–1
stadiometer 55–6
standard giving set 110, 159–61
stepping-stone (for addition) 18–19
straight-line graph 124–5
subtraction
    of multiples of ten, hundred, thousand 17
    mental strategies 15, 18–24, 104
    written methods 25–6
surface area 156
syringe 59, 61, 84, 85, 97, 102, 199

temperature 76–8, 89, 91, 125, 186–9,
    196–7
tenths, hundredths, thousandths 4, 7–12, 37,
    53, 93, 101, 137, 141
top-heavy fraction 134, 136
trailing zero (in decimals) 4, 38, 74, 79, 105
two-by-two array (for proportion) 149–55,
    159, 204

variables
    in a formula 124–5, 129, 188, 190–1
    in a population 85, 194–6
    in a proportional relationship 147–50,
        152, 208
volume
    abbreviations for units 60–61
    conversion of units 61–2
    imperial units 119
    litres and millilitres 59, 60, 62, 117
    reference items 59

weight
    abbreviations for units 68
    conversion of units 69–71
    distinction from mass 67
    imperial units 118–19
    reference items 67
    units met in healthcare 67
World Health Organization (WHO) 195

zero
    in number notation 3–6, 8–12, 37, 92–3
    in subtraction calculations 18, 21, 26
    in proportional variables 125
    ten to the power 3

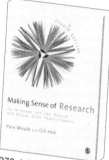
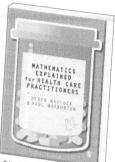
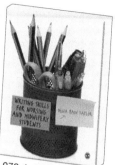
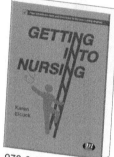
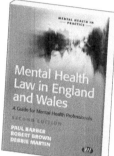
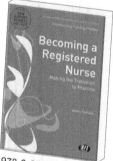
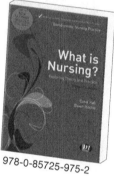
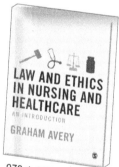
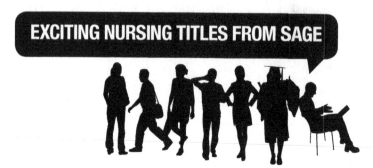